Ceramics in Orthopaedics

9th BIOLOX® Symposium
Proceedings

Edited by
JEAN-YVES LAZENNEC
MARTIN DIETRICH

Ceramics in Orthopaedics

JEAN-YVES LAZENNEC
MARTIN DIETRICH
Editors

Bioceramics in Joint Arthroplasty

9th BIOLOX® Symposium
Paris, March 26-27, 2004
Proceedings

with 127 Figures
and 12 Tables

STEINKOPFF DARMSTADT

ISBN 3-7985-1462-3 Steinkopff Verlag, Darmstadt

Cataloging-in-Publication Data applied for
A catalog record for this book is available from the Library of Congress.
Bibliographic information published by Die Deutsche Bibliothek
Die Deutsche Bibliothek lists this publication in the Deutsche Nationalbibliografie, detailed
bibliographic data is available in the Internet at <http://dnb.ddb.de>.

This work is subject to copyright. All rights are reserved, whether the whole or part of the
material is concerned, specifically the rights of translation, reprinting, reuse of illustrations,
recitation, broadcasting, reproduction on microfilm or in any other way, and storage in data
banks. Duplication of this publication or parts thereof is permitted only under the provisions
of the German Copyright Law of September 9, 1965, in its current version, and permission for
use must always be obtained from Steinkopff Verlag. Violations are liable for prosecution
under the German Copyright Law.

Steinkopff Verlag Darmstadt
a member of Springer Science+Business Media

http://www.steinkopff.springer.de

© Steinkopff Verlag, Darmstadt, 2004

The use of general descriptive names, registered names, trademarks, etc. in this publication
does not imply, even in the absence of a specific statement, that such names are exempt
from the relevant protective laws and regulations and therefore free for general use.

Product liability: the publishers cannot guarantee the accuracy of any information about
the application of operative techniques and medication contained in this book. In every
individual case the user must check such information by consulting the relevant literature.

Cover Design: TOP DESIGN, Thomas Schuster, Waiblingen

Production and Typesetting: druckerei justus kuch GmbH, Nürnberg

SPIN 10994726   105/7231-5 4 3 2 1 0 - Printed on acid-free paper.

Preface

**Dear Colleague and Participant
in Ceramics 2004 - 9ᵗʰ International BIOLOX® Symposium**

We are proud of the fact that once again we have been able to give you a copy of the proceedings of this symposium as a part of your registration materials. This is a major achievement that was only made possible by the excellent cooperation of the speakers, the publishing house and their staff and the Symposium Administrator and her staff. We would like to thank all of them for their hard work and dedication in meeting the tight deadlines required to make this a reality.

The proceedings of this symposium continue the on-going tradition of providing us with a valuable addition to our reference libraries. We hope that you will be pleased to receive this book, since within its covers, you will find the latest scientific and clinical information regarding the use of ceramics in orthopaedic surgery.

This is the first time that the symposium has taken place outside Germany. The reason we chose Paris, France, is obvious. It is because CeramTec has had a long and close relationship with the French orthopaedic community and because this community has been an incontestable pioneer in the use of ceramics in the field of orthopaedics. For these reasons it was only fitting to hold the symposium in the capital city of this much respected country of orthopaedic achievement. CeramTec is pleased that the University Hospital Pitié Salpétrière, our Honorary Presidents Prof. Sedel and Prof. Mittelmeier and our Symposium President, Prof. Lazennec have collaborated with us in the preparation and in the execution of **Ceramics 2004 - 9ᵗʰ International BIOLOX® Symposium**.

We hope that the quality of the presentations, the openness of the discussions, the efficiency of the organization, the knowledgeable participants and the City of Paris will have all worked together to make this a very special event in the pursuit of increased recognition of the benefits of our BIOLOX® ceramic technology by the Global Orthopedic Surgical community.

Jean-Yves Lazennec
Symposium President

Martin Dietrich
Managing Director
CeramTec Medical Products Division

List of contents

SESSION 3

Alternative Wear Couples Solutions/
Pro's and Con's

SESSION 4

Hip Revisions with Ceramic Solutions

SESSION 5

THR Instability and Dislocation: Different Solutions in THR

List of contributors and chairmen

FRANCESCO BENAZZO, Prof. Dr.
Università di Pavia Clinica Ortopedica
Via Taramelli 3
27100 Pavia, Italy

DANIEL J. BERRY, MD
Mayo Clinic
200 First Street SW
Rochester MN. 55905, USA

KURT BIDER
Centerpulse Orthopedics Ltd.
a Zimmer Company
P.O. Box
8404 Winterthur, Switzerland

BENJAMIN E. BIERBAUM, MD
New England Baptist Hospital
125 Parker Hill Avenue
Boston MA 02120, USA

MATTHIAS BLANKE
Dept. of Trauma Surgery
Erlangen-University
Krankenhausstr. 12
91054 Erlangen, Germany

MAX BÖHLER, Dr.
Herz Jesu Krankenhaus
Baumgasse 20 A
1030 Wien, Austria

JEAN-PIERRE BOURALY
Centerpulse France SA
127, Av. René Jacot - BP 81034 -
Technoland
25461 Etupes Cedex, France

PIERANGIOLA BRACCO, Dr.
Dipartimento di Chimica IFM dell'
Università di Torino
Via P. Giuria 7
10125 Torino, Italy

ELENA MARIA BRACH DEL PREVER, Dr.
Dipartimento di Traumatologia,
Ortopedia et Medicina del Lavoro dell'
Università di Torino
Via Zuretti 29
10126 Torino, Italy

WOLFGANG BURGER, Dr.
CeramTec AG
Fabrikstraße 23 - 29
73207 Plochingen, Germany

JACQUES CATON, Dr.
Clinique Emilie de Vialar - Chirurgie
Orthopédique et Réparatrice
116, rue Antoine-Charial
69003 Lyon, France

YVES CATONNÉ, Prof.
Hôpital Pitié Salpétrière -
Service de chirurgie
Orthopédique et Trauma
47-83, bd de l'Hôpital
75651 Paris Cedex13, France

ACHILLE CITTADINI, Prof.
Catholic University,
S.Cuore - Ist. di Patologia Generale
Largo F. Vito 1
00168 Roma, Italy

IAN CLARK, PhD
Loma Linda University Medical Center
Peterson Tribology Lab. Dept. of Orthopaedics
12340 Anderson St.
Loma Linda Ca 92350, USA

MICHELE CORBELLA, Dr.
Istituto Ortopedico Galeazzi
Via Riccardo Galeazzi, 4
20161 Milano, Italy

LUIGI COSTA, Prof.
Dipartimento di Chimica IFM dell'
Università di Torino
Via Giuria 7
10125 Torino, Italy

JEAN-PIERRE COURPIED, Prof.
Centre Hospitalo Universitaire
Cochin-Port Royal
27, rue due Faubourg St Jacques
75014 Paris, France

PAOLO DALLA PRIA, Ing.
Lima Lto spa
Via Nazionale
33038 Villanova di San Daniele
del Friuli (UD), Italy

MICHELE D'ANELLO, Dr.
1 Clinica Ortopedica Università di Bari
Piazza Giulio Cesare 11
70124 Bari, Italy

O. DE CAROLIS
1 Clinica Ortopedica Università di Bari
Piazza Giulio Cesare 11
70124 Bari, Italy

MASSIMO ESPOSITO, Dr.
Catholic University, Institute
of Orthopedics
Largo F. Vito 1
00168 Roma, Italy

P. FILIPPINI
Groupe Hospitalier Henri Mondor
Service d'Orthopédie
51, av. du Mal. De Lattre de Tassigny
94010 Créteil Cedex, France

JOHN FISHER, Prof.
School of Mechanical Engineering
University of Leeds Institute
of Medical and Biological Engineering
West Yorkshire
LS2 9JT Leeds, UK

JONATHAN P. GARINO, MD
University of Pennsylvania
3400 Spruce Street, Silverstein Two
Philadelphia, PA 19104-4283, USA

ROBERTO GIACOMETTI CERONI, Prof.
1st Ortop Galeazzi 4
Via R. Galeazzi 4
85112 Milano, Italy

SASCHA GOEBEL, Dr. med.
Dept. of Orthopaedics,
König-Ludwig-Haus,
Würzburg-University
Brettreichstr. 11
97074 Würzburg, Germany

VICTORIA GOOD
Smith & Nephew Orthopedics, Inc.
1450 Brooks Road
Memphis TN. 38116, USA

MOUSSA HAMADOUCHE, MD PhD
Centre Hospitalo-Universitaire
Cochin-Port Royal
27, rue due Faubourg St Jacques
75014 Paris, France

CHRISTIAN HENDRICH, Dr.
Universität Würzburg Orthop. Klinik
König-Ludwig-Haus
Brettreichstr. 11
97074 Würzburg, Germany

PHILIPPE HERNIGOU, Prof.
Groupe Hospitalier Henri Mondor
Service d'Orthopédie
51, av. du Mal. De Lattre de Tassigny
94010 Créteil Cedex, France

DAN HEUER
Smith & Nephew Orthopedics, Inc.
1450 Brooks Road
Memphis TN. 38116, USA

GORDON HUNTER, PhD
Smith & Nephew Orthopedics, Inc.
1450 Brooks Road
Memphis TN. 38116, USA

EILEEN INGHAM, Prof.
School of Biochemistry and
Molecular Biology University of Leeds
Leeds LS29JT, UK

GERARD M. INSLEY
Stryker Europe
Raheen Business Park
Limerik, Ireland

VOLKMAR JANSSON, Prof. Dr. med.
Ludwig-Maximilians-Universität
Orthopädische Klinik und Poliklinik
Marchioninistraße 15
81377 München, Germany

AN KAI NAN, PhD
Mayo Clinic
200 First Street SW
Rochester MN. 55905, USA

KRISTAPS J. KEGGI, MD
Keggi Orthopaedic Foundation –
Orthopaedic Surgery
1201 West Main St.
Waterbury CT 06708, USA

JOHN M. KEGGI, MD
Keggi Orthopaedic Foundation –
Orthopaedic Surgery
1201 West Main St.
Waterbury CT 06708, USA

ROBERT E. KENNON, MD
Joint Implant Surgery &
Research Foundation
17321 Buckthorn Dr.
Chagrin Fallls OH, 02120, USA

LUC KERBOULL, Dr.
Centre Hospitalo-Universitaire
Cochin-Port Royal
27, rue due Faubourg St Jacques
75014 Paris, France

MARCEL KERBOULL, Prof.
Centre Hospitalo-Universitaire
Cochin-Port Royal
27, rue due Faubourg St Jacques
75014 Paris, France

HEINO KIENAPFEL, Prof. Dr.
Klinikum der Philipps-Universität
Marburg Baldingerstraße
35033 Marburg, Germany

JEAN-YVES LAZENNEC, Prof.
Hôpital Pitié Salpétrière –
Service de chirurgie
Orthopédique et Trauma
47-83, bd de l'Hôpital
75651 Paris Cedex13, France

STEFAN LEYEN, Dipl. Ing.
CeramTec AG
Fabrikstraße 23 - 29
73207 Plochingen, Germany

GIULIO MACCAURO, Dr.
Catholic University,
Institute of Orthopedics
Largo F. Vito 1
00168 Roma, Italy

FOUZI MADI, Dr.
Hôpital Tenon - Chirurgie Orthopédique
4, rue de la Chine
75020 Paris, France

BERNARD MASSON, PhD
6, rue Eric Tabarly
31320 Pechabou, France

TIMOTHY MC TIGHE, PhD
Joint Implant Surgery & Research
Foundation
17321 Buckthorn Dr.
Chagrin Fallls OH, 44023, USA

ROLAND MEIZER, Dr.
Herz Jesu Krankenhaus
Baumgasse 20 A
1030 Wien, Austria

MICHAEL MENGE, Prof. Dr.
St- Marienkrankenhaus –
Orthopädische Abteilung
Salzburger Str. 15
67067 Ludwigshafen, Germany

Z. MERABET
Centerpulse France SA
127, Av. René Jacot
25461 Etupes Cedex, France

PATRICIE MERKERT, Dr.
CeramTec AG
Fabrikstraße 23 - 29
73207 Plochingen, Germany

HEINZ MITTELMEIER, Prof. Dr.
Universitätsklinik und Poliklinik
Homburg Saar
66421 Homburg/Saar, Germany

WOLFRAM MITTELMEIER, Prof.
Komm. Direktor der Klinik und Poliklinik für
Orthopädie, Universität Rostock
Ulmenstr. 44/45
18055 Rostock, Germany

FRANCESCO MURATORI, MD
Catholic University,
Institute of Orthopedics
Largo F. Vito 1
00168 Roma, Italy

STEPHEN B. MURPHY, MD
Center for Computer Assisted and
Reconstruction Surgery
125 Parker Hill Avenue, Suite 545
Boston MA., 02120, USA

JIM NEVELOS, Dr.
School of Mechanical Engineering
University of Leeds, Institute
of Medical and Biological Engineering
West Yorkshire
LS2 9JT Leeds, UK

RÉMY NIZARD, Prof.
Hôpital Lariboisière – Service d'Orthopédie
2, rue Ambroise Paré
75010 Paris, France

ALEXIS NOGIER
Groupe Hospitalier Henri Mondor
Service d'Orthopédie
51, av. du Mal. De Lattre de Tassigny
94010 Créteil Cedex, France

JUERG OEHY
Centerpulse Orthopedics Ltd.
a Zimmer Company
P.O. Box
8404 Winterthur, Switzerland

NORBERT PASSUTI, Prof.
CHU de Nantes- Hôpital Saint Jacques
Service de chirurgie orthopédique
Rue Saint Jacques
44035 Nantes, France

CORRADO PICONI, Prof.
Catholic University,
Institute of Orthopedics
Largo F. Vito 1
00168 Roma, Italy

HEINRICH PLANK, Prof., Dr. Ing.
ITV Denkendorf
Körschtalstraße 26
73770 Denkendorf, Germany

HANNS PLENK, Prof. Dr.
Institut für Biomaterialienforschung,
Histol.Embryol. Institut Univ. Wien
Schwarzpanierstraße 17
1090 Wien, Austria

A. POIGNARD
Groupe Hospitalier Henri Mondor
Service d'Orthopédie
51, av. du Mal. De Lattre de Tassigny
94010 Créteil Cedex, France

CHEN QINGSHAN
Mayo Clinic
200 First Street SW
Rochester MN. 55905, USA

LOTHAR RABENSEIFNER, Prof. Dr.
Klinikum Offenburg
Orthopädie und Orthopädische
Rheumatologie
Ebertplatz 12
77654 Offenburg, Germany

PATRICK REYNAUD, Dr.
Clinique Emilie de Vialar
Chirurgie Orthopédique et Réparatrice
116, rue Antoine-Charial
69003 Lyon, France

CLAUDE B. RIEKER, Dr.
Centerpulse Orthopedics Ltd.
a Zimmer Company
Sulzer Allee 8
8404 Winterthur, Switzerland

GÉRARD SAILLANT, Prof.
Hôpital Pitié Salpétrière
Chirurgie orthopédique et
traumatologique
47-83, bd de l'Hôpital
75651 Paris Cedex13, France

SERGIO SANGIORGI
ENEA -UTS Materials and Technology
Via Ravegnana, 186
48018 Faenza, Italy

LORENZO SCIALPI, Dr.
1 Clinica Ortopedica Università di Bari
Piazza Giulio Cesare 11
70124 Bari, Italy

LAURENT SEDEL, Prof.
Hôpital Lariboisière - Service d'Orthopédie
2, rue Ambroise Paré
75010 Paris, France

ALESSANDRO SGAMBATO
Catholic University,
Institute of Orthopedics
Largo F. Vito 1
00168 Roma, Italy

GIOVANNI SOLARINO, Prof.
1 Clinica Ortopedica Università di Bari
Piazza Giulio Cesare 11
70124 Bari, Italy

GIUSEPPE SOLARINO, Dr.
1 Clinica Ortopedica Università di Bari
Piazza Giulio Cesare 11
70124 Bari, Italy

TODD D. STEWART, Dr.
School of Mechanical Engineering
University of Leeds
Institute of Medical and
Biological Engineering
West Yorkshire
LS2 9JT Leeds, UK

ROBERT M. STREICHER
Stryker SA
Florastrasse 13
8800 Thalwil, Switzerland

NICOLA TARTAGLIA, Dr.
1 Clinica Ortopedica Università di Bari
Piazza Giulio Cesare 11
70124 Bari, Italy

JOANNE L. TIPPER, Dr.
School of Mechanical Engineering
University of Leeds Institute
of Medical and Biological Engineering
West Yorkshire
LS2 9JT Leeds, UK

STEFANIE VETTER, Dipl. Ing.
Wasgaustr. 32
67065 Ludwigshafen, Germany

KIRSTIN WIDDING
Smith & Nephew Orthopedics, Inc.
1450 Brooks Road
Memphis TN. 38116, USA

LUIGI ZAGRA, Dr.
Divisione Istituto Ortopedico Galeazzi
Via R. Galeazzi 4
85112 Milano, Italy

SESSION 1

Long Term Clinical Experience with Ceramic Components

1.1 Ceramic on Ceramic Bearings Used with Proximal Modular Stems in THA

K. J. Keggi, J. M. Keggi, R. E. Kennon and T. McTighe

Abstract

Introduction: Osteolysis generated by wear debris remains a problem in total hip arthroplasty. Alternate bearings surfaces are sought in an attempt to reduce debris particles and prolong prosthetic wear.

Ceramic on ceramic surfaces have a long clinical history but have encountered a number of problems due to design and material properties. Impingement with malposition of the components, ceramic chipping, and ceramic fractures with malposition of the acetabular component have been problems.

Material: This paper will review 185 ceramic on ceramic bearings used with proximal modular stem designs. Two different stem designs and four different cup designs all utilizing ceramic heads and ceramic inserts manufactured by CeramTec were used.

Conclusion: The recent development of proximal femoral modular stem designs provides better surgical exposure and improved orientation of the prosthetic components. This will reduce the complications due to ceramic implants.

Introduction

The senior authors (KJK, JMK) have performed over 800 ceramic on ceramic total hip arthroplasties at our institution since 1983. Demand for durability, better fit, and greater surgical options has led to the use of newer modular designs in recent years, including nearly 200 modular total hip replacements utilizing ceramic on ceramic interfaces. While early ceramic materials with monoblock designs suffered from ceramic chipping, ceramic fractures with malposition of the acetabular components, and impingement with malposition of the components, it has been our experience and impression that newer modular designs have provided better surgical exposure, improved orientation of the components, and greater flexibility in restoration of normal biomechanics. This has in turn reduced the complications due to ceramic implants and obviated the need for extra long skirted ceramic heads.

Materials and Methods

Medical records were retrospectively reviewed for all patients undergoing primary total hip arthroplasty utilizing both modular designs and ceramic on ceramic interfaces. No patients were excluded from this group. All operations were performed using the modified anterior approach developed by the senior surgeon [1]. Specific parameters examined included demographic data, stem type, acetabular type, and nonmedical complications related to the prosthesis or surgical technique, such as dislocation, malposition, subsidence, fracture, or damage to the ceramic component.

Two proximal modular stem designs were utilized in this series. The first is the Apex Modular™ Hip Stem shown in Figure 1 (Apex Surgical, LLC, Lakeville, MA). The second is the PROFEMUR™ Z stem shown in Figure 2 (Wright Medical Technology, Inc., Arlington, TN). Four acetabular components were used: the LINEAGE® acetabular system (Wright Medical Technology), the TRANSCEND® acetabular system (Wright Medical Technology), the BICON-PLUS® acetabular system (PLUS Orthopedics, San Diego, CA), and the Cer-Met™ acetabular system (Apex Surgical).

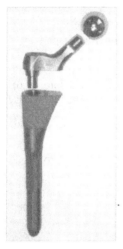
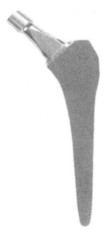

Figure 1:
Apex Modular™ Hip Stem
(Apex Surgical, LLC, Lakeville, MA).

Figure 2:
PROFEMUR™ Z stem (Wright Medical
Technology, Inc., Arlington, TN).

This data is shown in Table 1 and was comprised of 185 total hip replacements.

Femoral Component	Acetabular Component	Total
Apex	Lineage	64
	Transcend	23
	Cer-Met	55
	Bicon	2
ProFemur Z	Lineage	23
	Transcend	5
	Cer-Met	11
	Bicon	2
TOTAL		**185**

Table 1:
Summary of all modular ceramic on ceramic THA performed.

Results

Five nonmedical complications were noted in this series of 185 total hip replacements, including two hip dislocations, one acetabular component dislocation, one femoral fracture with stem subsidence, and one failed ceramic acetabular liner. The average length of follow-up was approximately two years, but thus far all four complications that have occurred were apparent within six weeks of the initial surgery. The summary of nonmedical complications is presented in Table 2.

Femoral Component	Acetabular Component	Complication
ProFemur Z	Transcend	Ceramic liner fracture at 6 weeks post-op; atraumatic, changed liner/shell/neck/head
ProFemur Z	Cer-Met	Dislocated at 6 weeks post-op and required closed reduction with no further problems
Apex	Bicon	Dislocated with 6 weeks post-op & required open reduction, components retained. [Patient later sustained fractured femur in MVA vs. pedestrian accident and underwent ORIF.]
Apex	Lineage	Acetabular component dislocated at 1 week; underwent acetabular and femoral head replacement at that time. Previous sciatic nerve palsy pre-operatively after acetabular ORIF (MVA) likely contributed. (See Figure 3).
Apex	Cer-Met	Unappreciated femoral fracture discovered at 6 weeks with component subsidence; converted to Echelon cemented stem.

Table 2:
Summary of nonmedical complications.

The first represented the only failure of the ceramic materials in this series. The patient noted the new onset of pain for one week without recalled antecedent trauma approximately six weeks after undergoing primary total hip arthroplasty with a ProFemur Z stem and Transcend cup with ceramic liner. Evaluation revealed him to have a cracked ceramic liner. It is impossible to state the cause of this fracture; it could be due to pure ceramic materials failure or it may have been an undetected malalignment of the component within its titanium shell. The patient underwent exchange of the liner, acetabular shell, neck, and femoral head without further problems. The modular design proved advantageous in this instance, facilitating modular component exchange.

The second complication was a hip dislocation six weeks post-operatively that was associated with noncompliance with total hip precautions. This patient had undergone a primary THA with a ProFemur Z femoral stem and Cer-Met acetabular component. After undergoing a closed reduction under anesthesia, the patient had no further problems after a year of follow-up.

The third complication involved a patient who underwent primary THA with an Apex femoral stem and a Bicon acetabular component. This patient sustained a dislocation six weeks from the time of surgery after being noncompliant with total hip precautions and required open reduction of the hip with components retained. The patient did well for a limited period of follow-up until suffering extensive trauma as a pedestrian struck by a motor vehicle in which he sustained a periprosthetic femur fracture but no ceramic failure despite his trauma.

The fourth complication was an acetabular dislocation in a patient with a failed traumatic acetabular fracture ORIF (Figure 3a). It occurred one week post-operatively after primary total hip arthroplasty. This patient had an Apex femoral stem and a Lineage acetabular component. Contributing factors were pre-existing sciatic nerve palsy with foot drop, her post-traumatic acetabular bone deficiency, obesity, and active hyperextension of the hip. The revision was relatively easy since it was possible to remove the proximal (modular) neck component and achieve acetabular exposure without removal of the entire femoral prosthesis (Figure 3b). The patient's THA subsequently has remained stable.

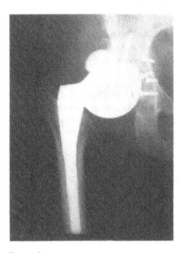

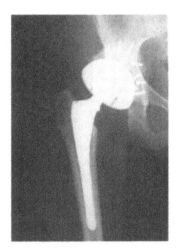

Figure 3a:
Acetabular component dislocation.

Figure 3b:
Post-operative film after acetabular and femoral head replacement.

The fifth complication occurred with an Apex stem and Cer-Met acetabular component in which a peri-operative femur fracture was unappreciated at the time of surgery. This was subsequently noted six weeks post-operatively with subsidence of the femoral component that necessitated its revision to a cemented Smith-Nephew-Richards (Memphis, TN) EchelonTM femoral stem.

Discussion

Since Pierre Boutin attempted the first ceramic total hip arthroplasty in 1970, there has been interest in ceramic bearing surfaces to improve implant longevity and decrease wear [2]. However, early experience with ceramics indicated high failure rates due to component loosening and early need for revision, with failure rates approaching 27% - 35% in some studies [3,4,5]. Our own early results using the noncemented Autophor were satisfactory and matched the success of Mittelmeier, and we have had some extremely good long term successes with the device in some young and very active patients [6,7,8]. We have not seen any osteolysis on long term follow-up, but the overall failure rate has been unsatisfactory because of inadequate acetabular fixation, acetabular migration, fractures of the thinner acetabulums, and inadequate osteointegration of the femoral component [9].

Although many investigators concluded that much of the fault with these prostheses lay with design and technique in greater part than the ceramic material, ceramic on ceramic joints were abandoned in the United States for over a decade. Ceramic heads in polyethylene acetabular components continued to be used in the United States while the ceramic itself was improved (Biolox-Forte) and its fixation to bone modified in Europe. While first generation ceramics before 1985 had fracture rates as high as 10% in some reports [10], contemporary third generation alumina ceramics have smaller grain size, fewer impurities, and a more stable crystalline structure with fracture rates as low as 4 in 100,000 [11].

Prosthetic designs have also improved with enhancements such as highly polished articular surfaces, optimized clearance between the head and liner to provide a fluid boundary, improved sphericity, tightened tolerances for tapers, and elimination of skirts on ceramic heads. The advent of modular femoral components has also facilitated the insertion and positioning of the ceramic joint itself. A decrease in malaligned acetabulums and femoral necks should optimize long term wear of the ceramics.

The marriage of contemporary ceramic articulating surfaces and proximal modular design affords several benefits. Modular designs allow better surgical exposure, and modularity allows multiple sizing and positioning options to improve orientation of the implants and, ultimately, the stability and biomechanical restoration of the hip replacement. Current designs also do not require the extra long skirted ceramic heads which have historically been more likely to impinge and break.

Our current series of modular ceramic on ceramic hip replacements has shown promising results after an average of one year of follow-up. While this is still an early period of observation, it is our impression that these hip replacement systems perform well and offer a significant addition to the surgeon's armamentarium.

Conclusion

While ceramic on ceramic surfaces have a long clinical history with progressive improvement in materials science, a relatively new approach has been the implantation of ceramic on ceramic surfaces with proximal modular total hip designs. In reviewing all of our modular ceramic on ceramic total hip replacements, we have found them to have excellent performance with few problems in the short term. In particular, there was only a single failure due to chipping or fracture of the ceramic materials – one acetabular liner – and no failures of the ceramic femoral heads. It is our impression that newer modular total hip designs utilizing ceramic interfaces have reduced the complications which were present in earlier monoblock femoral prostheses utilized 15 to 20 years ago. Modular femoral components also allow better surgical exposure, improved component orientation, and reproduction of the proximal femoral anatomical variations such as varus, valgus, or anteversion.

References

1. Light TR, Keggi KJ. Anterior approach to hip arthroplasty. Clin Orthop 152:255, 1980.
2. Boutin P, Arthroplastie Totale de Hanche par Prosthes en Alumine Fritte, Rev Chir Orthop, Vol. 58:229-246, 1972.
3. O'Leary J., et al, Mittelmeier Ceramic Total Hip Arthroplasty, J Arthroplasty, Vol.3:87-96, 1988.
4. Mahoney O., et al, Unsatisfactory Results with a Ceramic Total Hip Prosthesis, JBJS, Vol. 72-A:6623-671, 1990.
5. Winter M, et al. Ten to 14 year results of a ceramic hip prosthesis. Clin Orthop, 282: 73-79, 1991.
6. Mittelmeier H, Heisel J. Sixteen years of experience with ceramic hip prostheses. Clin Orthop 282: 64-72, 1992.
7. Hoffinger SA, Keggi KJ, et al. Primary ceramic hip replacement: A prospective study of 119 Hips. Orthopedics. 14(5):523-31, 1991.
8. Huo MH, Martin RP, Zatorski LE, Keggi KJ. Total hip replacement using the ceramic Mittelmeier prosthesis. Clin Orthop 332:143-150, 1996.
9. DiCaprio M, Huo MH, Keggi JM, et al. Ceramic-on-ceramic articulation in cementless THAs done in young patients: a 10-year follow-up study. Program and abstracts of the American Academy of Orthopaedic Surgeons 69th Annual Meeting; February 13-17, 2002; Dallas, Texas. Paper 170
10. Toni A, et al. Ceramics in total hip arthroplasty. P1501-44. In: Wise DL, et al. (eds): Encyclopedic Handbook of Biomaterials and Bioengineering. Marcel Dekker Inc.; New York, 1995.
11. Willmann G. Ceramic Ball Head Retrieval Data, Reliability and Long-Term Results of Ceramics in Orthopaedics: 4th International CeramTec Symposium, 62-63, 1999.
12. Garino J. Ceramic-on-Ceramic Total Hip Replacements: Back to the Future, Orthopedic Special Edition, Vol. 6 No. 1:41-43:2000.

1.2 Surface Analysis of Explanted Alumina-Alumina Bearings

G. M. Insley and R. M. Streicher

Abstract

The purpose of this study was to characterize wear stripes on explanted third generation ceramic-on-ceramic components. Macroscopy, light microscopy and scanning electron microscopy (SEM) was carried on the wear stripes to determine their extent and the material failure mechanism that led to their formation. The analysis shows that the wear stripes were formed through high stress, point contact of the head on the rim of the cup. This type of damage occurs due to microseparation of the head and cup during specific patient activities.

Introduction

Alumina ceramic-on-ceramic articulation is one of the best choices for hip joint bearings for young and active patients. Their low wear, less than 0.5 mm^3 per 10^6 cycles in vitro and the benign periprosthetic tissue reaction to the small amount of debris produced make them an ideal biomaterial for this application [1-3]. Even though the normal wear mechanism of these bearings is generally understood to be slight relief polishing; recently a number of wear stripes were reported on a series of explanted alumina-on-alumina components [4, 5]. The ceramics components concerned were part of a larger series of more than 1,500 successful implants done by mainly one surgeon at the Orthopaedic Hospital Sydney, Australia. The majority of the bearings were removed during a routine re-operation for a variety of clinical conditions such as psoas tendonitis, periprosthetic fracture and infection. The surgeon noticed that the surface of the heads had a slight loss of polish in some areas and this coincided with a similar mark on the cup. This is the first time that wear stripes of this type have been reported on modern third generation alumina components. The objective of this study was to characterize the wear stripes in terms of their extent and the material failure mechanism that led to their formation. This data will further add to the baseline of knowledge about ceramic articulation for artificial implants and will be essential in validating simulator testing for ceramic-on-ceramic components.

Materials and Methods

Sixteen explanted alumina-alumina couples were analysed in this study. Eleven components had evidence of wear stripes (11 heads and 8 liners). The remaining components, which showed no wear stripes, were used as controls.

Macro examination involved recording dimensional and angular measurements of the stripes and correlating the data with the available clinical information:
On the heads, the length of the stripes and their maximum width, the latitude angle of the centre of the stripe relative to the head equator ('inclination' angle,

see figure 1 (a)) and the angle of the long axis of the scar to a line of latitude running through the centre of the scar ('tilt' angle, see figure 1 (b)) were measured.

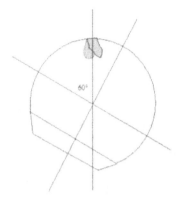

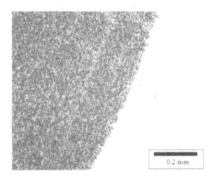

Figure 1a:
Latitude angle of stripe.

Figure 1b:
Tilt angle of stripe.

On the cups, the circumferential length of the stripes and their maximum width were measured in each case.

For examination at higher magnification, a conventional optical microscope was used. Various lenses were used to image the stripes. For scanning electron microscopy, a number of representative samples were chosen. The heads were mounted on the SEM stub using graphite adhesive, and the area of interest was lightly sputter-coated with gold/palladium to provide conductivity.

Results and Discussion

The following features appeared to be common to all explanted heads and cups showing localised wear stripes:

The worn areas on the heads are usually well defined with sharp boundaries, especially at the ends and on the trunnion side of the stripe, see figure 2(a) and (b). There tended to be more damage outside the main stripe on the pole side than on the trunnion side, see figure 2(b).

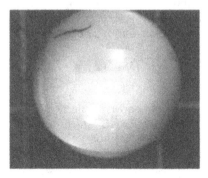

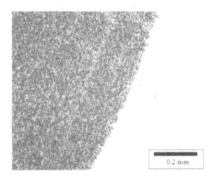

Figure 2a:
Macrograph of stripe on alumina head.

Figure 2b:
Micrograph of well-defined boundary.

The worn areas on the cups were lens-shaped, generally narrower than on the matching head, and were usually located along the 'blend' line between the highly polished hemispherical bearing surface and the less well-polished convexly curved chamfer near the cup edge, see figure 2(c). In a number of cases, it was apparent that a very narrow stripe existed over an extended length of the blend line outside the main lens-shaped stripe, in one or both directions. In extreme cases, the stripe was found to extend beyond this convexly curved region onto the conical chamfer region, along the outer blend line, see figure 2(d).

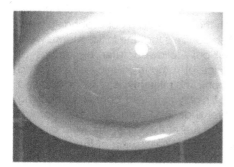
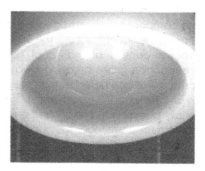

Figure 2c:
Macrograph of narrow stripe.

Figure 2d:
Macrograph of narrow stripe.

The lengths of the worn areas on the head and cup are similar, and increase in size with implantation time, suggesting that the initial non-conforming contact of the head on the cup rim becomes conforming with time and/or number of cycles of movement.

Both heads and cups exhibited scratches in the form of lines of pits both within and outside the main stripe areas. Scratches were most prevalent on components with more pronounced stripes. These could be parallel to the length of the stripes, and/or at a steep angle across them. They were often in parallel sets.

There was a wide variation in the tilt angle of the scar to the lines of latitude on the head. Generally, the direction correlated with whether the implant was on the patient's left or right side. All stripes showed a tilt direction that was retroverted, i.e. tilting backwards in respect to the body. There was also a wide variation in inclination angle of the head stripes to the head equator, from 0° to 60°.

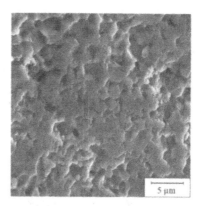

Figure 3:
Head stripe centre region showing grain pull-out.

The SEM analysis of the wear stripes showed that they all comprised of grain pull-out with clear facetted sides to the remaining pits. In some cases, there was evidence of subsequent smoothing over of the surface, almost a partial re-polishing of the surface, with some fine-scale debris being trapped in the pits, see figure 3.

Conclusions

Out of the sixteen explants examined, eleven showed evidence of wear stripes. The components examined with a stripe on the head had a corresponding wear scar on the rim of the cup. The SEM analysis confirms that the initial intense wear process consists of individual grain 'pull-out' followed later by groups of unsupported grains breaking away. Evidence of some repolishing of the pitted surface was also noted at high magnifications. This pitting type of wear, followed by a later smoothing process, is typical of highly localized contacts occurring initially between the head and cup rim over a defined area. As these contacts conform geometrically with increments in the size of the stripe, the wear process becomes less severe and can even lead to partial repolishing of the damaged surface.

In conclusion, the wear scars examined on these explanted alumina-alumina couples were formed through high stress, point contact of the head on the rim of the cup. This, coupled with a lack of lubrication at this point initiated the reported wear stripes without leading to either catastrophic failure or super-critical wear values. This type of contact occurs, in vivo, through microseparation of the head and cup and this mechanism needs to be incorporated into modern simulator testing of alumina-on-alumina components and also other hard-on-hard bearings.

Acknowledgements

The authors wish to acknowledge the staff and technicians at the National Physical laboratory for their contribution and assistance in this work and William L. and K. Walter (Sydney Northside Orthopedic Surgeons) for samples and discussions.

References

1. Amstutz, H. C., Campbell, P., Kossovsky, N. and Clarke, I. C.: Clin. Orthop. Vol. 276 (1992), p.7.
2. Maloney, W. J., Jasty, M. and Harris, W. H.: J. Bone and Joint Surg. Vol. 72B (1990), p.966.
3. Schmalzreid, T. P., Jasty, M. and Harris W. H.: J. Bone and Joint Surg. Vol.74 (1992), p.849.
4. Nevelos, J. E., Ingham, E., Doyle, C., Streicher, R., Nevelos, A. B., Walter, W. and Fisher, J.: J. Arthro. Vol.15 (2000), p.793.
5. Stewart, T. Tipper, J., Streicher, R., Ingham, E. and Fisher, J.: J. Mater. Sci. (In Press).

1.3 A Ten Years Experience with Alumina-Alumina Hip Replacement

G. Solarino, L. Scialpi, M. D'Anello, N. Tartaglia, O. De Carolis and G. B. Solarino

Introduction

Polyethylene wear, due to a cascade of events activated from macrophages, is the main reason of bone resorption and periprosthetic osteolysis and usually takes to the failure of the implant.

This has pushed bioengineers to research new materials to reduce friction, wear and tissutal reaction: considering that nowadays many younger and younger people are operated of hip arthroplasty with higher mechanical and functional requests, the target of research is to increase longevity of implants.

Since sixties, Sir John Charnely, the father of modern hip arthroplasty surgery, had already realized that ceramic had a low friction coefficient, foreseeing its use in the future when technology would have been able to produce better ceramics for biological use.

In fact, ceramics with its low friction resistance, with its high hydrophilic properties, with its particular hardness and considering its low reaction to its wear debris, could be the best bearing surface for hip arthroplasty.

The surgical technique needs to be optimal and precise and components geometry needs to respect cinematic and articular biomechanical theories.

The alumina-alumina replacement is agree with *Low-Frictional Torque Arthroplasty* theories of Sir J. Charnely who announced that frictional torque (M_t) occurring between two components is directly proportional to the head diameter (D), to the articular charge (W) and to the friction coefficient between components (μ).

$$M_t = \mu WD/2$$

The friction coefficient of Alumina-Alumina replacement ($\mu_{ce/ce}= 0{,}035$) is about three times less than the one of Metal-Polyethylene ($\mu_{me/pe} = 0{,}1$): this means that to have the same frictional torque value of Metal-Polyethylene replacement of 22,25 mm, we could use a 67 mm head articulating within an acetabular diameter 2 mm larger.

Materials and Methods

Nowadays in the $I^\wedge$ Clinica Ortopedica of University in Bari (Italy), in patiens who need a biological fixation, we use mainly the Cerafit M cup manufacted by Ceraver Osteal (Roissy, France).

The press-fit cementelss titanium shell consisted of a pure titanium core with a titanium alloy mesh to allow bone ingrowth: its design consisted of an hemispherical shape with a flattening in the polar region and circumferential gutters (Triradius Cup). For these reasons the cup is inserted in 2 mm underreamed acetabulum. There are 3 holes: 2 for additional screw fixation and 1 on the apex for the peg of the liner which is held in the metal back by a conical sleeving and combined with a 32 mm alumina femoral head.

From January 1994 to April 2003, 121 consecutive alumina-alumina hip replacement in 74 females and 47 males were performed. The median age of patients at the time of surgery was 58 (range 25-74 years). The initial diseases inducing hip replacement were: primary coxarthrosis in 67 (55,4%) hips, atraumatic avascular necrosis in 26 (21,5%), fracture of the upper femur in 18 (14.9%), coxarthrosis after hip dysplasia in 8 (6.6%), rheumatoid arthritis in 2 (1.6%). All the operations were primary procedures, performed or supervised by the senior author (G.B.S.).

Two additional screws have been used in 19 cases (15.7 %).

Three different stems were used: a cemented collared smooth anodized Ti stem in 40 cases (33%), two cementless (one anatomical and one HA-coated straight, fig. 1) Ti stems in 81 cases (67%).

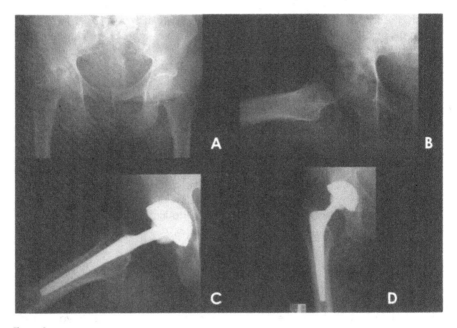

Figure 1:
Pre-operative AP and axial x-ray; C-D: X-ray control at a 36 months follow-up.

Results

98 hips (81%) have been reviewed at an average follow-up of 41 months: 92 (93.8%) have showed no clinical and/or radiological signs of impending failure (Fig. 2), 6 (6.2%) had undergone a revision (2 infections, 2 sinking of the anatomical cementless stems, 1 stem fracture, 1 recurrent dislocation).

None of the implants have been revised due to mechanical failure of the ceramic components.

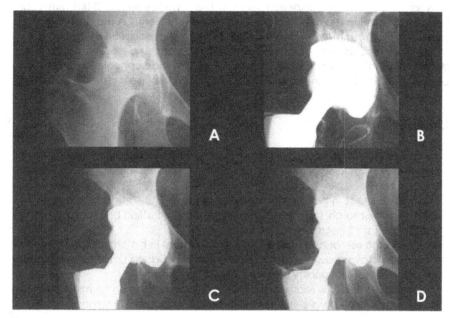

Figure 2:
Alumina-alumina 32 mm cementless implant in avascular necrosis. A: Pre-operative x-ray;
B: Post-operative x-ray; C: X-ray control at a 12 months follow-up; D: The X-ray control at a 8
years follow-up shows optimal osteointegration.

Discussion

Alumina-alumina hip replacement have been firstly used from French and
German surgeons in the early seventies.

Boutin used alumina cups directly fixed in the acetabular bone or using methyl-
methacrylate, leading to a different stiffness in the implant-host system and so
producing mobilization of the cup from the bone.

The Mittlemeier system gave troubles with both biological fixation of a alumina
screwed-in cup and "mushroom-shaped" heads: this realized easily an
impingement of the skirt against the acetabular component giving the chipping
and breakage of one ceramic components.

The use, in new acetabular prosthetic designs, of a metal-back (often in
Titanium with a porous external surface) represents a shock absorber that
reduces the different stiffness between ceramic and bone.

The abandon of skirted heads and the improvement in surgical procedures
reduce the impingement risks.

With 32 mm heads used nowadays, resistance to the fracture of materials is
increased very much, passing from 38 KN of seventies to the 89 KN: this value is
almost the double of the one (46 KN) indicated from the American FDA as a
minimal burst strength limit.

A 32 mm head improves both mechanical performance and grants a wider
articular range of movement than the one possible with a 28 mm head (8°-10°
more, using a 12-14 mm cone).

Wear tests and clinical experiences show linear wear values of 0,001 mm/year in alumina-alumina replacement: this is 200 times smaller than the one of metal-polyethylene (0,1 mm/year) and it explains the drastic reduction of debris.

The biocompatibility of ceramic is demonstrated by the peculiar reaction to its debris, with main presence of fibroblasts, minimal of macrophages and absence of giant-cells, and so by the almost complete absence of periprosthetic osteolysis.

Conclusions

In last years, many improvements on quality of hip arthroplasty materials have been made, especially for sphericity, circularity, insert-head clearance, prosthetic stem and cone.

Anyway it is recommended to use products from the same manufactory, to avoid risk of "mismatch" between components and/or fretting phenomena at the cone-head or shell-insert interfaces.

Worries in the use of alumina-alumina replacement in hip arthroplasty have to be considered over-passed considering studies that suggest us better and better results for mechanical quality and longevity of implants.

According to this, it is reasonable to admit that alumina on alumina bearing surface seems to be a valid alternative in the hip replacement surgery.

References

1. Bizot P et al - Alumina-on-Alumina Total Hip Prostheses in Patients 40 Years of Age or Younger, CORR, 379:68-76, 2000
2. Bizot P et al - Press-fit Metal Backed Alumina Sockets. A Minimum 5-Year Follow-up Study, CORR, 379:134-142, 2000
3. Boutin P – Arthroplastie totale de hance par prothese en alumine frittee, Rev Chir Orthop 58;229-46, 1972
4. Charnley J – Low Friction Arthroplasty of the Hip. Theory and Practice. Springer-Verlag,, Berlin, Heidelberg, New York, 1979
5. Clohisy JC and Harris WH – The Harris-Galante porous-coated acetabular component with screw fixation. An average ten-year follow-up study, JBJS 81A (1), 66-73, 1999
6. Fisher J, Ingham E, Stone MH – Alternative bearing couples in total hip replacements: solutions for young patients. Hip International, Vol. 13, n.1 (suppl.2) pp. S31-S35, 2003
7. Garino JP – Ceramic-Ceramic total hip Replacement : Intraoperative Considerations – Bioceramics in Joint Arthroplasty, edited by Aldo Toni and Gerd Willmann – Proceedings 6th International BIOLOX Symposium, March 23/24, 2001
8. Mendes DG et al – Ten rules of Technique for ceramic bearing surfaces in total hip arthroplasty – Bioceramics in Hip Joint Replacement, edited by Gerd Willmann and Karl Zweymüller – Proceedings 5th International CeramTec Symposium, Febr. 18/19, 2000.
9. Mittelmeier H – Zementlose Verankerung von Endoprothesen nach dem Tragrippen-prinzip. Z. Orthop. 112: 27-33, 1977
10. Pitto RP et al – Clinical outcome and quantitative evaluation of periprosthetic bone-remodeling of an uncemented femoral component with taper design. A prospective study, Chir Organi Mov. Apr-Jun;86(2):87-97, 2001
11. Prudhommeaux F et al – Analysis of Wear Behavior of Al/Al Hip Prosthesis after 10 years of implantation, in Legeros RZ and Legeros JP eds: Proceedings of the 11th International Symposium on Ceramics in Medicine, 1998
12. Sedel L et al – Alumina -Alumina Hip Replacement in Patients Younger than 50 years old, CORR, 298:175-183, 1994

1.4 Thirty Years Experience with all Ceramic Bearings

L. Sedel

Introduction

To overcome the problem of foreign body reactions to polyethylene debris generated by sliding couple in total hip replacement, we did implant since 1977 an alumina (Al_2O_3) against alumina bearings total hip prosthesis.

The first alumina-on-alumina total hip arthroplasty was implanted in April 1970 by the French surgeon Pierre Boutin. Until 1977, the alumina head was either glued with an epoxy resin or screwed to the femoral stem. However, this method of fixation led to an unacceptable rate of head to stem dissociation, with forty-five cases of 791 (5.7%) hip replacements performed between 1970 to 1977. Moreover, the quality of the alumina ceramic was non-optimal with large grain size and broad grain size distribution, combined with a low purity. All these adverse factors were responsible for ten fractures of the alumina components (six heads and four sockets) of 791 hip replacements (1.3%). Notable progresses were made in 1976 with the introduction of a Morse taper locking mechanism of the alumina head to the titanium stem, together with an improvement in the material manufacturing process, leading to the production of surgical grade dense alumina ceramic. At this time we introduced a new stem design made of titanium alloy smooth and covered with a layer of 5000A° of titanium oxide. The stem was designed to be cemented but also to fill the medullary canal resulting in a thin cement mantle; The idea came from the adverse results obtained with the regular small Charnley stem. We introduced the first alumina on alumina prosthesis in 1977.

The French experience was followed by Mittelmeier, Griss, and Heimke in Germany, Furuya in Japan, Pizziferato in Italy, and Salzer in Austria.

Over this 30 years period a lot of datas were documented concerning tissues reaction , in vivo wear behaviour, fractures, and clinical outcome.

Tissues reactions were documented on animal studies and on histological sections of tissues retrieved during revision procedure. Alumina debris were few appeared as yellow dots of 0,5m in diameter. Usually pure fibrocytic reactions were noticed except when the prosthesis has been loosed for many months or years resulting in massive foreign body reaction related to the amount of mix debris of metal, cement and ceramic. PGE2 studies on retrieved tissues comparing those around metal on polyethylene sliding couple found less production than around ceramic on ceramic sliding. This is in accordance to other laboratory works from I. Catelas or J. Fisher who demonstrated less inflammatory reaction with this couple than with other combinations.

Cementless plain alumina socket was documented after natural death of the patient who had this prosthesis implanted for 12 years. There was no direct bone to alumina contact but fibrous tissues and the bone did enter into alumina grooves resulting in some type of interlocking which explains the good results of this device.

Ceramic materials retrieved at revision were analysed. Sphericity, surface roughness, wear volume were plotted against quality of alumina grain size. There was a correlation between these parameters: old alumina did wear more than more recent one. In some occasion wear was as low as some microns for a 15 years period in use. This is two thousand times less than a regular metal on polyethylene sliding couple. and 100 times less than a metal on metal prosthesis.

Fracture mechanism is related to crack propagation into the material; This is diminished by using a high quality alumina with high density, high purity, low porosity and small grain size randomly distributed. This has been obtained by improving the manufacturing processes and by applying High Isostatic Pressure (HIP) technique. During the first period fracture rate was in the range of 2%. Then it drops to less than 0,1 %. We suspect the current fracture rate to be in the order of 0,05% for a ten year period of use. Cone technology is also highly relevant and a failure in this technology either at the femur or at the socket level may explain some recent fractures. In our clinical experience we have recently published 13 fractures of an alumina component over a 25 years period. and more than 5500 prosthesis with at least one alumina material implanted. Majority of these events could be easily explained by some mistakes either in component size, cone technology or material quality. Few fractures could not be explained; Even of concern, these events are extremely lo, easy to revise if recognised quickly and have to be compared to the major advantages of this material which authorize a full activity including sports or strenuous activities even in young age and active population. The results we did publish in this population clearly demonstrated these advantages over periods up to 20 years.

Clinical outcome

More than 3500 total hips in selected young and /or active patients were implanted. Many publications concerned this topic. The more recent one concerned a series implanted by P.Boutin in PAU during the year 1980. One hundred and eighteen hips in 106 patients were operated. Mean age was 62 years. There was different fixation systems. Cemented socket in 85 cementless socket in 23 cemented stem in 89 cementless stem in 19.

At the twenty-year follow-up evaluation, forty-five patients (fifty-one hips) were still alive and had not been revised, twenty-five patients (twenty-five hips) had undergone revision of either or both components, twenty-seven patients (thirty hips) had died from unrelated causes, and nine patients (twelve hips) were lost to follow-up. The mean Merle d'Aubigné hip score was 16.2 ± 1.8 at the latest follow-up. Survival of the cup at twenty years with revision for any reason as the end-point was 85.6 percent (95 percent interval confidence, 72.2 to 99.0 percent) for cementless cups versus 61.2 percent (95 percent interval confidence, 46.8 to 75.6 percent) for cemented cups, respectively. Survival of the stem at twenty years with revision for any reason as the end-point was 84.9 percent (95 percent interval confidence, 71.1 to 98.8 percent) for cementless stems versus 87.3 (95 percent interval confidence, 77.4 to 97.1 percent) for cemented stems. Wear of the prosthetic components was undetectable on plain radiographs. Periprosthetic cystic or scalloped lesions were recorded in three of the 118 hips. No fracture of the alumina socket or head was recorded.

Another study concerned a more recent design of the socket which consisted in a metal back titanium alloy shell covered with a pure titanium mesh with an alumina liner. From 1990 to 1992 71 hybrid alumina on alumina hip replacements were performed in 71 hips (62 patients) with a mean age of 46 years at surgery. The nine year survival rate was 93% if revision for any cause was the end point and 98,4% if revision for aseptic loosening was the end point. One socket had a complete radiolucent line less than 1 mm thick. There was no component migration nor osteolysis.

It was clear from this long term experience that the weak part was the socket fixation; New systems including metal back alumina with press fit shell covered with a titanium mesh was efficient; We modified it 6 years ago to a rough titanium surface covered with hydroxyapatite. This is our current material which as far as we observe solve the problem.

Since 1997 we moved also to a cementless stem with an identical surface.

Conclusion

31 years experience of this material allows us to draw some firm conclusion; This alumina on alumina bearing system is safe if the material if of high quality, if cone technology is accurate and if the material has a significant thickness. It gives interesting results without any physical limitation specially in young and active patients. Revision is easy due to the lack of foreign body reaction. Concerned are still represented by some risk of fracture and by the cost. Surgical technique is also highly relevant because this material is not as friendly for users as the regular plastic. But long term expectancy without revision may be considered when these aspects are considered.

References

1. PRUDHOMMEAUX F., HAMADOUCHE M., NEVELOS J., DOYLE C., MEUNIER A., SEDEL L. Wear of alumina-alumina total hip arthroplasties at a mean 11-year follow-up. Clin. Orthop,379,113-122,2000
2. SEDEL L, NIZARD R, BIZOT P, MEUNIER A, BLANQUAERT D, WITVOET J. Evolution of alumina-alumina implants: a review. Clin Orthop, 379,48-54,2000
3. BIZOT P, NIZARD R, LARROUY M, WITVOET J, SEDEL L. Press fit metal backed alumina sockets: a minimum 5 years follow up study Clin Orthop. 379,134-142 ,2000
4. BIZOT P, BANALLEC L, SEDEL L NIZARD R,. Alumina on alumina total hip prostheses in patients 40 years of age or younger Clin Orthop. 379,68-76,2000
5. HAMADOUCHE M, SEDEL L.,Ceramics in Orthopaedics, J Bone Joint B, 2000, 1095-1099
6. HAMADOUCHE M, Boutin P, Daussange J, Bolander M, and Sedel L. Alumina-on-Alumina Total Hip Arthroplasty: A Minimum 18.5-Year Follow-up Study. Journal of Bone and Joint Surgery 84A(1): 69-77, 2002.
7. HANNOUCHE Didier MD, Nich Christophe MD, Bizot Pascal MD, Meunier Alain PhD; Nizard Rémi MD, PhD, Sedel Laurent MD: CERAMIC BEARINGS FRACTURES: HISTORY AND PRESENT STATUS. Clin orthop and rel. res dec 2003.
8. SEDEL L, CABANELA M, Hip surgery materials and developments, Dunitz London 1999.

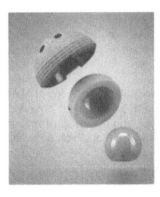

Figure 1:
Metal back alumina socket with an alumina liner.
32 mm head.

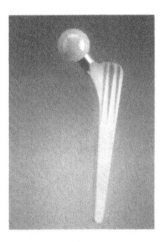

Figure 2:
Cementless stem fully coated HA.

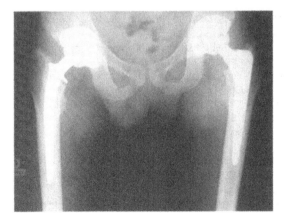

Figure 3:
Bilateral total hip in a 17 years old boy for severe avascular necrosis of the femoral head, 3 years follow up. No pain, can perform some type of physical activities without any limitation.

1.5 Ceramic/Ceramic Total Hip Replacement: The American Experience with Stryker Implants

B. E. Bierbaum
J. D'Antonio, W. Capello, M. Manley and R. Deshmukh

Abstract

A major challenge for total hip arthroplasty is to minimize wear and osteolysis in young, active patients. Alumina ceramic bearings have shown superior wear resistance and lubrication and do not carry the risk of ion release. In a prospective randomized study (ABC), 514 hips were implanted. All patients (average age, 53 years) received the same press-fit hydroxyapatite coated femoral stem; two thirds (345 hips) received alumina ceramic bearings, and one third (169 hips) received a cobalt-chrome–on–polyethylene bearing. A fourth arm (Trident) was included involving use of a metal-backed acetabular component implanted in 209 patients. At a mean follow-up of 35.2 months (range, 24-48 months), there was no significant difference in clinical performance between the patient cohorts. The cohort of patients included in the ABC, Trident, and extended access portion of the study represents a population of 2313 patients with no device related failures attributable to the ceramic on ceramic articulation used in these patients. This new experience involves the use of improved ceramic materials and new design considerations that eliminate the risks and complications of past experiences with ceramic implants and provides a safe bearing option for young patients.

Introduction

Advances in implant design and materials and improvements in surgical technique and instrumentation have made total hip arthroplasty (THA) one of the most durable and successful treatments in medicine [1]. Reproducible high-quality results are attained regularly, with survivorship commonly lasting ≥10 to 15 years [2]. The success of this procedure has allowed expansion into a wider, younger and more active patient population [3]. As THA is used in younger and higher demand patients and as life expectancies increase, the orthopaedic community continually is seeking new methods and materials that may extend the useful life of THAs. The challenge today is to develop new bearing surfaces that can function at a high level and prolong the life of well-fixed implants.

Past experiences with alumina ceramic bearings have been met with disappointing results because of increased component loosening, ceramic component fracture, and isolated examples of accelerated wear of the bearing surface [4]. One objective of this clinical study was to evaluate the use of alumina-on-alumina ceramics with proven implants that have had successful track records with regard to fixation (on a prospective randomized basis). These results were compared with the results of cobalt-chrome–on–polyethylene bearings, which is the current standard for THA. A second objective of this study was to compare the complications that are related directly to the alumina iceramic bearing couple with the complications that were seen with previous designs in the 1970s and 1980s.

Materials and Methods

In October 1996, a U.S. IDE prospective randomized study began comparing alumina-on-alumina ceramic bearings with cobalt-chrome–on–polyethylene bearings. Patient enrollment was completed in October 1998, after 514 hips were implanted in 458 patients. A total of 22 investigators at 16 sites participated in this investigational device exemption (IDE) study (see Appendix 1). Approval by the Food and Drug Administration of the protocol and patient informed consent were obtained before study initiation. Each site was required to submit the protocol with consent to the hospital institutional review board. The consent explained that the study was randomized and that the patient would receive the control or the investigational ceramic device based on a randomization scheme, and the patient agreed to participate in the study before determination of which device they would receive. Neither the patient nor the surgeon was aware of the device that was selected randomly for implantation.

There were 3 arms to the study that included 3 cup designs; 2 had alumina-on-alumina bearings (systems 1 and 2), and 1 had the control of cobalt-chrome–on–polyethylene (system 3) (Fig. 1).

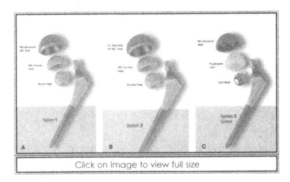

Click on image to view full size

Figure 1:
(A) Porous-coated acetabular shell, alumina ceramic acetabular insert, alumina ceramic femoral head, and hydroxyapatite (HA)-coated titanium femoral stem.
(B) Titanium arc deposited HA-coated acetabular shell, alumina ceramic acetabular insert, alumina ceramic femoral head, and HA-coated titanium femoral stem.
(C) Titanium porous-coated acetabular shell, polyethylene acetabular insert, cobalt-chrome femoral head (ion bombarded), and HA-coated titanium femoral stem.

All patients received the same femoral stem (Omnifit HA; Howmedica Osteonics, Allendale, NJ). There was a one-third chance of receiving 1 of the 3 cup designs and a two-thirds chance of receiving an alumina-on-alumina bearing surface. System 1 comprised a porous-coated titanium shell and an Alumina Bearing Couple (ABC; Stryker Howmedica Osteonics, Allendale, NJ) insert. System 2 had an arc deposited titanium shell with hydroxyapatite coating and an ABC insert. System 3, the control group, had a porous-coated titanium shell and a polyethylene insert. All of the cups had a peripheral self-locking design with a 1-mm increased peripheral radius over the radius of the dome of the socket. The diameter of head size and the inside diameter of acetabular inserts are outlined in Table 1.

Table 1:
Comparison of femoral head size.

Head Size (mm)	ABC Alumina Components Trident		
	Control Cobalt-Chrome Femoral Heads		
26	NA		
	NA		
	20 (12.1%)		
28	35 (10.0%)		
	1 (1%)		
	136 (82.4%)		
32	314 (90.0%)		
	74 (69%)		
	9 (5.5%)		
36	NA		
	32 (30%)		
	NA		
Abbreviation: NA - not applicable.			

Acetabular components of 32-mm inside diameter and alumina ceramic femoral heads were available for implants that were ≥50 mm in diameter. Most (136 cases [82.4%]) of the control implants had 28-mm inside diameter polyethylene inserts and 28-mm cobalt-chrome femoral heads implanted to avoid the potential for increased volumetric polyethylene wear that could occur with the routine use of 32-mm diameter femoral heads. It was believed at the time of the study design that the routine use of 32-mm head size against polyethylene potentially would bias the study against the control group and in favor of the alumina couple, for which the use of 32-mm heads was not an issue.

In the initial study involving 349 ABC alumina ceramic implants, no component fracture was experienced. Nine peripheral chips occurred with the ABC system because of technical problems involving placement of the alumina ceramic insert within the titanium acetabular component. If the ABC shell is canted and wedged in the shell and an impaction force to seat the insert subsequently is delivered, a peripheral chip can occur. After recognizing this technical problem, a fourth study arm (Trident implant; Howmedica Osteonics, Allendale, NJ) was instituted evaluating a metal-backed alumina insert that is placed within the acetabular shell. The alumina ceramic insert of the Trident system has been assembled with a shrink-fit titanium sleeve on the outside that mates with a peripheral taper lock within the acetabular shell. The equatorial edge of the metal sleeve extends past the ceramic liner to prevent articulation of the femoral taper with the ceramic surface. This titanium sleeve also protects the rim of the alumina ceramic from chipping on insertion and increases the burst strength of the alumina ceramic [24]. Six centers from the original ABC study and five additional ones (see Appendix 2) inserted 209 of these implants in a prospective nonrandomized study using system 3 as a control.

The demographics for the combined ABC and Trident study are shown in Table 2.

Table 2:
Patient demographics ABC and Trident Study.

	ABC System 1 ABC System 2 Trident Control
No. cases	172 177 209 165
No. of patients	163 171 194 161
Male/female(%)	66/34 64/36 66/34 60/40
Mean age (y)	. 53 53 52 53
Mean weight (lb)	187.7 191.8 189.7 188.5
Mean height (in)	68.6 68.6 68.4 68.4
Length of follow-up (mo)	47.7 47.6 30.7 46.6
Diagnosis (%)	
OA	81% 76% 81% 76%
PTA	2% 5% 3% 5%
AVN	14% 18% 11% 16%
Other	3% 1% 4.5% 3%

Abbreviations: OA - osteoarthritis; PTA - post-traumatic arthritis; AVN - avascular necrosis; No - number.

The follow-up included 349 alumina-on-alumina hips (318 patients), with 335 hips (307 patients) at 24 months, 243 hips (227 patients) at 36 months, and 72 hips (71 patients) at 48 months (mean, 35.2 months' follow-up). For the 165 hips (161 patients) included in the control group, follow-up included 149 hips (147 patients) at 24 months, 111 hips (111 patients) at 36 months, and 26 hips (26 patients) at 48 months (mean, 33.6 months' follow-up). All groups had a preponderance of males (60-66%), a young mean age of 52 to 53 years, and a predominant diagnosis of osteoarthritis (76-81%). All patients in all study groups suffered from noninflammatory disabling arthritis.

Data coordinators collected radiographic and clinical data preoperatively, early postoperatively (6-8 weeks), at 6 months, at 1 year, and at 1-year intervals thereafter. The level of pain and functional parameters, including distance the patient could walk, stair climbing, need for external support, sitting, limp, and participation in recreational activities were evaluated at each visit, and a composite Harris hip score (HHS) was calculated for each patient [5]. The postoperative radiographs were evaluated by an orthopaedic surgeon who was not part of the investigator group. Anteroposterior and lateral radiographs of the patients were obtained at each visit. The postoperative radiographs were evaluated for radiolucencies, implant fixation, implant migration, and erosion of cortical bone (osteolysis). The acetabulum was divided into 3 zones based on DeLee and Charnley [6], and femoral components were evaluated using Gruen zones 1 through 14 [7]. Component stability was determined using the criteria described by Engh et al [8].

Results

Clinical data for the ABC system with minimum 2-year follow-up are shown in Table 3.

Table 3:
Clinical data.

	ABC System 1 (2-4 y; mean, 3 y) (n = 166) ABC System 2 (2-4 y; mean, 3 y) (n = 172) Trident (2-3 y; mean, 2.5 y) (n = 193) Control (2-4 y; mean, 3 y) (n = 151)
Pain none/slight (%)	91 92 94 93
Limp none/mild (%)	98 96 99 97
Mean Harris hip score	95.4 96.6 97.2 95.9

Harris % G/E (%)	94
	94
	97
	96
Patient satisfaction ("Are you satisfied with results?") (%)	95
	98
	97
	97

Abbreviation: G/E, Good/Excellent scoring for the Harris hip score. G = Harris hip score of 80-89 and E = Harris hip score of 90-100.

Complications for the ABC and Trident groups are reported in Table 4.

Table 4:
Complications.

Complication	System 1
	System 2
	Trident
	Control
Revision	
Acetabular	0
	1 (0.6%)
	1 (0.5%)
	2 (1.2%)
Femoral	1 (0.6%)
	0
	1 (0.5%)
	2 (1.2%)
Both	1 (0.6%)
	2 (1.1%)
	0
	0
Insert and/or head only	0
	0
	2 (1.0%)
	5 (3.0%)
Deep Joint Infection	1 (0.6%)
	1 (0.6%)
	0
	2 (1.2%)
Intra op Fem Fx	6 (3.5%)
	7 (4.0%)
	4 (1.9%)
	7 (4.2%)

Postoperative femoral fracture	5 (2.9%)
	2 (1.1%)
	1 (0.5%)
	2 (1.2%)
Dislocation	4 (2.3%)
	6 (3.4%)
	4 (1.9%)
	7 (4.2%)
Heterotopic bone	6 (3.5%)
	7 (4.0%)
	8 (3.8%)
	10 (6.1%)
Intraoperative insert chip	5 (2.9%)
	4 (2.3%)
	0
	NA
Abbreviation: NA - not applicable	

Four (1.2%) revisions have taken place for the entire study group (349 cases) implanted with alumina ceramic bearings, 1 in system 1 and 3 in system 2. Eight revisions were reported in the control group (system 3). In ABC systems 1 and 2, 1 revision of the femoral stem and head was for postoperative femoral fracture; 1 revision of the acetabular component, insert, and head was for recurrent dislocation; 1 revision of all components was for sepsis; and 1 revision of all components was for suspected, but not confirmed sepsis. For the cobalt-chrome–on–polyethylene control group, 1 revision of the stem and head was for postoperative femoral fracture; 1 revision of the stem and head was for leg-length discrepancy; 1 revision of the acetabular shell insert and head with retention of the femoral component was for acute sepsis; 1 revision of the acetabular shell, head, and insert was for loosening of the acetabular component; and 4 revisions of the insert and head were for recurrent dislocations. Peripheral chips (2.6%) occurred in 9 hips of the ABC alumina ceramic study group at the time of insertion. In all but 1 case, the alumina ceramic liner or shell or both were replaced. In 1 hip, the chipped insert was seated, impacted, and left in place without any known secondary complications. No complications have been reported related to these events in these 9 cases, and none of the revised cases had insertional chips. No alumina ceramic fractures or bearing surface–related failures have occurred in the 318 patients (349 hips) who received the ABC alumina ceramic bearing inserts.

Mean composite Harris hip scores for all ABC groups were consistently >90 out of 100 points (excellent range). At a mean 3 years postoperatively, the mean composite Harris hip scores for the ABC systems 1, 2, and 3 were 95.4 (158 hips), 96.6 (163 hips), and 95.9 (142 hips). Patients were asked if they were satisfied with the results of the surgery at each follow-up evaluation. At a mean 3 years postoperatively, patient satisfaction with the surgery was reported as 95% (157 hips), 98% (169 hips) and 97% (145 hips) with ABC systems 1, 2, and 3.

In evaluating revisions in the Trident study arm, one case involved revision of the femoral stem and head due to post-op femoral fracture which occurred at the 7 week postoperative visit as the patient descended from the exam table. One acetabular component, Trident insert, and alumina head were revised approximately 9 months postoperatively to an all-polyethylene cup with a 32 +5mm head due to acetabular component loosening. In one instance of chronic instability, the acetabular insert only was revised 19 months postoperatively to a Trident Crossfire polyethylene insert. Another case involved subluxation and led to revision of the acetabular insert and head at 22 months postoperatively.

Table 5 provides a summary of the radiographic results of the ABC and Trident study arms.

Table 5:
Radiographic results.

Radiographic Parameter	System 1 (2-4 y, mean, 3 y) (n = 162) System 2 (2-4 y; mean, 3 y) (n = 169) Trident (1-3; mean, 2 y) (n = 185) Control (2-4; mean, 3 y) (n = 149)
Femoral RLL zone 1	8 (6.0%) 3 (2.3%) 4 (2.3%) 11 (8.8%)
Femoral RLL zone 7	2 (1.5%) 1 (0.8%) 0 1 (0.8%)
Stem subsidence	0 1 (0.8%)* 0 0
Unstable stem fixation	1 (0.8%) 1 (0.8%)* 0 1 (0.8%)
Acetabular RLL	
Zone 1	10 (6.2%) 1 (0.6%) 1 (0.5%) 10 (6.7%)
Zone 2	3 (1.9%) 0 0 7 (4.7%)

Zone 3	25 (15.4%)
	0
	6 (3.3%)
	35 (23.5%)
Acetabular RLL	
3 Zone	0
	0
	0
	2 (1.6%)
Acetabular shell migration	1 (0.7%)
	0
	0
	1 (0.8%)*†
Unstable acetabular component	2 (1.5%)
	0
	0
	3 (2.4%)†
Abbreviation: RLL - radiolucent line. * Same femoral component. † Same acetabular component.	

One case (0.6%), implanted with ABC system 2, was reported to have an unstable femoral component. The same case was reported to have femoral subsidence. The investigator reported that the patient fell, and a postoperative femoral fracture was suspected, although it was not evident on radiographs. The patient has not been revised at this time. Two cases (systems 1 and 3) were reported to have unstable acetabular components. One case (system 1– microstructured surface treatment) was determined to have radiographic evidence of the acetabular shell loosening with radiolucent lines in zones 1 and 3 on evaluation of the 3-year radiographs. The patient is asymptomatic at this time. One case implanted with control system 3 was reported to have shell migration at the 3-year radiographic review. The patient is pending revision of a loose acetabular component. No cases of acetabular loosening were reported for system 2, which has an arc deposited titanium surface with hydroxyapatite treatment. At a minimum 2-year follow-up for 169 cases evaluated for ABC system 2, only 1 cup (0.6%) exhibited a radiolucent line in any zone. This case was reported to have a 1-mm radiolucent line in zone 1 at 2 years postoperatively. For the 162 cases evaluated for ABC system 1, 33 cups (20.4%) exhibited a radiolucent line in any zone, and 25 cups (15.4%) were reported as having a radiolucent line in zone 3. For the 149 cases evaluated for control system 3, 45 cups (30.2%) exhibited a radiolucent line in any zone, and 35 cups (23.5%) were reported as having a radiolucent line in zone 3. No hip was reported to have radiolucencies in all 3 acetabular zones (Fig. 2).

Critical evaluation of the Trident arm of the study With a 1- to 3-year follow-up, this study group has performed from a clinical standpoint equal to systems 1, 2, and 3. There have been no peripheral chips because of the protective metal backing of the Trident, and there have been no ceramic fracture or ceramic bearing surface–related failures.

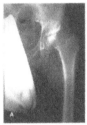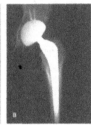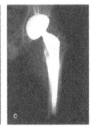

Figure 2A-C:
A 41-year-old laborer with Perthes's disease and secondary degenerative joint disease. Anteroposterior radiographs of (A) preoperative, (B) 6-week postoperative, and (C) 4-year postoperative views.

Discussion

In the 1970s and 1980s, emphasis was placed on achieving a high degree of fixation for THAs. In the 1990s, it became obvious that a major challenge to long-term success was to minimize wear and osteolysis. The most common mode of long-term failure for THA is aseptic loosening, and it has been recognized that particulate debris, in particular, polyethylene particulate debris, is responsible in many cases for the inflammatory response that leads to bone resorption and loosening of the implants over time [9-14]. Many patients are undergoing reoperation without revision of components in the form of liner or head exchange with or without bone grafting secondary to osteolytic periprosthetic bone loss. The actual biologic event is caused by macrophage-induced resorption of bone at the prosthesis–bone interface secondary to the presence of particulate polyethylene debris [15,16]. If the life expectancy of implants is to be improved significantly, better bearing surface materials are needed for the future.

Two approaches are being pursued simultaneously to minimize wear of THA bearing surfaces. The alternatives to traditional metal-on-polyethylene include improved cross-linked polyethylene components and hard-on-hard bearings, including metal-on-metal and alumina-on-alumina ceramic. Although new cross-linked polyethylene components offer great hope for reduced wear, long-term follow-up is necessary to determine their true potential for long-term success. With regard to hard-on-hard bearings, of the 2 alternatives, metal-on-metal versus alumina-on-alumina ceramic, the alumina ceramic bearing couples have several theoretical advantages. One is the elimination of polyethylene. Retrievals from alumina-on-alumina ceramic implants have indicated that alumina ceramic debris is less biologically reactive than particulate metal or polyethylene debris [17-20]. The extremely low coefficient of friction and superior wear resistance of alumina ceramics promises wear rates that are appreciably less than those of polyethylene-on-metal and metal-on-metal couples [11,17,20]. Alumina ceramics are extremely hard, scratch resistant, and stable at high temperatures, and their hydrophilic nature provides for improved lubrication over other bearing surfaces [21]. Alumina ceramic bearings have no potential for ion release, a distinct advantage over metal-on-metal couplings. However, Alumina-on-alumina ceramic bearings have their own unique limitations, such as higher rigidity, the consequences for neck-socket impingement, the potential for fracture, and a history of early loosening revealed in previous clinical experiences reported from Europe and the United States [4,22,23]. As a result of these complications and past experiences, the alumina ceramic materials and prosthetic designs have evolved and improved.

Contemporary alumina ceramic material is of higher quality than earlier alumina ceramics. As a result of hot isostatic pressing, currently used alumina ceramics are produced with a dense fine grain alumina with a grain size <2 μ and limited grain boundaries and inclusions. The grain size of these materials has been reduced for Biolox material (CeramTec, Plochingen, Germany) from a high of 4.2 μm in 1984 to 1.8 μm for Biolox forte in 1995. Corresponding to the reduction in grain size, burst strength has increased from 46 kN in 1984 to 65 kN in 1995 [24]. Minimal Food and Drug Administration standards for burst strength for alumina ceramic components are 46 kN and no failures at 20 kN. These material improvements have increased greatly the toughness and strength of alumina ceramics. High tolerances for mating of the alumina ceramic to the implant have been established, eliminating a major cause for stress risers and fractures that occurred in the past [24]. Laser etching instead of mechanical engraving is used now, which minimizes stress risers. Proof testing also has been introduced. All modern components are subjected to a burst strength examination before sterilization and shipping [25,27]. Current alumina ceramic bearing implants benefit from the advantages gained as a result of improvements in the preparation of the alumina ceramics and new design features, such as improved manufacturing tolerances for mating of the alumina ceramics to the implants. Also, the alumina ceramic bearings now are used with femoral stems and acetabular components that have had a successful track record with regard to fixation. These combined improvements provide for a new approach to alumina-on-alumina ceramic bearings and hold great promise for prolonged fixation of implants, particularly in young and more active patients.

The clinical experience in Europe with alumina-on-alumina ceramic acetabular components began in 1970. Clinical experience in the United States began in the early 1980s with the introduction of the Autophor and Xenophor devices (threaded alumina ceramic cup designs developed by Mittelmeier in Europe) (Smith & Nephew, Richards, Memphis, TN). These ceramic-on-ceramic devices had disappointing results primarily because of design issues [4]. The primary design concerns were neck socket impingement, which could lead to femoral neck wear, cup rim fracture, debris degeneration, and loosening [17]. The use of these implants in the United States eventually was abandoned. Although these were alumina ceramic bearings, device failures were in large part design related rather than material related [4]. The implants that were used in the early 1980s were inferior to today's designs with regard to achieving lasting fixation and to mating of the alumina ceramic to the implants. The goal of current ceramic-on-ceramic components is to resolve design and fixation limitations and deficiencies revealed in earlier ceramic-on-ceramic designs.

An important feature of the ABC system is the protection of the alumina ceramic acetabular liner from impingement on the femoral neck. The components used in this study are recessed within the metal shell, avoiding the possibility of impingement on the periphery of the alumina ceramic, which can lead to chipping and fracture. Perhaps the greatest concern with the use of alumina ceramics today is the issue of fracture. A review of the literature reveals a progressive decline in the incidence of component fractures as the quality of alumina ceramic materials improves with continued use of alumina ceramic bearings in Europe [22,25]. A report published in 1995 on the use of alumina ceramic femoral heads in the United States indicated a fracture rate of 1.9% in 4 of the189 alumina ceramic femoral heads used. All alumina ceramic heads fractured within the first 2 years after implantation [23]. These femoral heads were used on femoral stems that were manufactured in the hospital, and there was a mismatch between the alumina ceramic femoral head and the trunnion of the femoral stem. This is an important issue, which has been resolved by appropriate design modifications. Precise matching of the taper-locking interface between the alumina ceramic and femoral or acetabular components is crucial to minimize the risk of stress risers and fracture. A recall of zirconium femoral heads (St. Gobain, Cedex, France) occurred because of reported fractures. The alumina femoral heads used in this study (ABC system) are of a completely different composition, are produced by a different manufacturer (CeramTec), and have not experienced a fracture.

To date, >7,000 ABC implants have been implanted in Europe and Australia. Two fractures of the acetabular liner have been reported. In both cases, the components intentionally were left in a canted nonseated position. Both of these implants failed through fracture in a short period. When an acetabular component of the ABC design is fully seated and when a femoral component from these systems is fully seated on a clean and appropriate trunnion, the risk of fracture is estimated to be 1 in 20,000 [24]. The risk of fracture of a metal component used in THA has been reported to be 27 in 10,000 [26].

Critical evaluation of the Trident arm of the study demonstrates that with a 1- to 3-year follow-up, this study group has performed from a clinical standpoint equal to systems 1, 2, and 3. There have been no peripheral chips because of the protective metal backing of the Trident, and there have been no ceramic fracture or ceramic bearing surface–related failures. The cohort of patients included in the ABC, Trident, and extended access portion of the study represents a population of 2313 patients with no device related failures attributable to the ceramic on ceramic articulation used in these patients.

Combining advances in material and design provides for a new approach to alumina-on-alumina ceramic bearings that hold great promise for increasing durability of implant fixation, particularly in young, active patients (Fig. 2). By combining new, high-quality alumina ceramic acetabular and femoral bearing heads with THA systems that have achieved long-term stable fixation, we believe a substantial increase in the fixation longevity of implants can be achieved. Current alumina-on-alumina ceramic bearing systems feature high-quality, fine grain alumina ceramic heads and inserts and hip stems and acetabular shells with clinically established successful fixation histories. We believe the use of alumina-on-alumina ceramic bearings, when properly designed, is indicated for younger and more active patients.

References

1. Papatheofanis F: Technology report: prosthetic hip and knee arthroplasty. University Hospital Consortium (UHC) Technology Advancement Center, Oakbrook, IL, 1994

2. Black J: Prospects for alternate bearing surfaces in total replacement arthroplasty of the hip. In: Proceedings of the 2nd Symposium on Ceramic Wear Couple, Stuttgart, Germany, 1997

3. Capello WN, D'Antonio JA, Feinberg JR, et al: Hydroxyapatite-coated total hip femoral components in patients less than fifty years old: clinical and radiographic results after five to eight years of follow-up. J Bone Joint Surg Am 79:1023, 1997

4. Mahoney OM, Dimon JH: Unsatisfactory results with a ceramic total hip prosthesis. J Bone Joint Surg Am 72:663, 1990

5. Harris WH: Traumatic arthritis of the hip after dislocation and acetabular fractures: treatment by mold arthroplasty: an end result study using a new method of result evaluation. J Bone Joint Surg Am 51:737, 1969

6. DeLee JG, Charnley J: Radiological demarcation of cemented sockets in total hip replacement. Clin Orthop 121:20, 1976

7. Gruen TA, McNeice GM, Amstutz HC: Modes of failure of cemented stem-type femoral components: a radiographic analysis of loosening. Clin Orthop 141:17, 1979

8. Engh CA, Massin P, Suthers KE: Roentgenographic assessment of the biologic fixation of porous-surfaced femoral components. Clin Orthop 257:107, 1990

9. Dumbleton J: Wear and prosthetic joints. Churchill Livingstone, New York, 1991

10. National Institute of Health: Total hip replacement. NIH Consensus Statement 1994. 12(5):1, 1994

11. Saikko VO, Paavolainen PO, Slatis PS: Wear of the polyethylene acetabular cup, metallic and ceramic heads compared in a hip simulator. Acta Orthop Scand 64:391, 1993

12. Harris WH: Osteolysis and particle disease in hip replacement. Acta Orthop Scand 65:113, 1994

13. Geesink R, Hoefnagels N: Six-year results of hydroxyapatite-coated total hip replacement. J Bone Joint Surg Br 77:534, 1995

14. Schmalzried T, Kwong L, Jasty M: Periprosthetic bone loss in total hip arthroplasty: the role of polyethylene wear debris and the concept of the effective joint space. J Bone Joint Surg Am 74:849, 1992

15. Goldring SR, Schiller AL, Roelke M, et al: The synovial-like membrane at the bone-cement interface in loose total hip replacements and its proposed role in bone lysis. J Bone Joint Surg Am 65:575, 1983

16. Shanbhag AS, Jacobs JJ, Glant TT, et al: Composition and morphology of wear debris in failed uncemented total hip replacement. J Bone Joint Surg Br 76:60, 1994

17. Clarke IC: Role of ceramic implants: design and clinical success with total hip prosthetic ceramic-to-ceramic bearings. Clin Orthop 282:19, 1992

18. Sedel L, Kerboull L, Christel P, et al: Alumina-on-alumina hip replacement: results of survivorship in young patients. J Bone Joint Surg Br 72:658, 1990

19. Lerouge S, Huk O, Yahia LH, et al: Ceramic-ceramic and metal-polyethylene total hip replacements: comparison of pseudomembranes after loosening. J Bone Joint Surg Br 79:135, 1997

20. Fisher J, Besong AA, Firkins PJ, et al: Comparative wear debris generation in UHMWPE on ceramic metal on metal and ceramic on ceramic hip prostheses. Presented at 46th Annual Meeting, Orthopaedic Research Society, Orlando, FL, 2000

21. Skinner HB: Ceramic bearing surfaces. Clin Orthop 369:83, 1999

22. Fritsch E, Gleitz M: Ceramic femoral head fractures in total hip arthroplasty. Clin Orthop 328:129, 1996

23. Callaway GH, Flynn W, Ranawat C: Case report: fracture of the femoral head after ceramic-on-polyethylene total hip arthroplasty. J Arthroplasty 10:855, 1995MEDLINE

24. Willmann G: Ceramic ball retrieval data. In: Proceedings of the 4th Symposium on Ceramic Wear Couple, Stuttgart, Germany, 1999

25. Heros RJ, Willmann G: Ceramics in total hip arthroplasty: history, mechanical properties, clinical results, and current manufacturing state of the art. Semin Arthroplasty 9:114, 1998

26. Heck DA, Partridge CM, Reuben JD, et al: Prosthetic component failures in hip arthroplasty surgery. J Arthroplasty 10:575, 1995MEDLINE

27. Guarino J: Ceramic-on-ceramic total hip replacements: back to the future. Orthopedic Special Edition 6, 2000

APPENDIX 1

Investigators and Co-Investigators in the ABC Study (Excluding Authors)

Paul Pongor, MD, New England Baptist Hospital, Boston, MA
Edward Hellman, MD, Orthopaedics of Indianapolis, Indianapolis, IN
Clifford W. Colwell, MD, Scripps Clinic, LaJolla, CA
Steven Copp, MD, Scripps Clinic, LaJolla, CA
Richard Walker, MD, Scripps Clinic, LaJolla, CA
Joseph H. Dimon, III, MD, Peachtree Orthopaedic Clinic, Atlanta, GA
John D. Henry, MD, Peachtree Orthopaedic Clinic, Atlanta, GA
Jonathan Hottenstein, MD, Sewickley Valley Hospital, Moon Township, PA
William Hozack, MD, Rothman Institute, Philadelphia, PA
William L. Jaffe, MD, Hospital for Joint Diseases, Orthopedic Institute, New York, NY
Paul DiCesare, MD, Hospital for Joint Diseases, Orthopedic Institute, New York, NY
Patrick Meere, MD, Hospital for Joint Diseases, Orthopedic Institute, New York, NY
Ormonde Mahoney, MD, Athens Orthopedic Clinic, PA, Athens, GA
Kenneth E. Marks, MD, Cleveland Clinic Foundation, Cleveland, OH
J. Wesley Mesko, MD, Ingham Medical Center, Lansing, MI
James R. Roberson, MD, Emory Sports Medicine & Spine Center, Decauter, GA
Sean P. Scully, MD, PhD, Duke University, Durham, NC
Scott Siverhus, MD, Flower Hospital, Sylvania, OH
Robert Zann, MD, Boca Raton Hospital, Boca Raton, FL

APPENDIX 2

Investigators and Co-Investigators in the Trident Study (Excluding Authors)

Joseph McCarthy, MD, New England Baptist Hospital, Boston, MA
Arnold Scheller, MD, New England Baptist Hospital, Boston, MA
Donald Reilly, MD, New England Baptist Hospital, Boston, MA
Jonathan Hottenstein, MD, Sewickley Valley Hospital, Moon Township, PA
James R. Roberson, MD, Emory Sports Medicine & Spine Center, Decauter, GA
Scott Siverhus, MD, Flower Hospital, Sylvania, OH
Robert Zann, MD, Boca Raton Hospital, Boca Raton, FL
William Hozack, MD, Rothman Institute, Philadelphia, PA
William L. Jaffe, MD, Hospital for Joint Diseases, Orthopedic Institute, New York, NY
Patrick Meere, MD, Hospital for Joint Diseases, Orthopedic Institute, New York, NY
Ormonde Mahoney, MD, Athens Orthopedic Clinic, PA, Athens, GA
Clifford W. Colwell, MD, Scripps Clinic, LaJolla, CA
Richard Walker, MD, Scripps Clinic, LaJolla, CA
Steven Copp, MD, Scripps Clinic, LaJolla, CA
J. Wesley Mesko, MD, Ingham Medical Center, Lansing, MI

1.6 Results Obtained for 474 Cementless Hip Endo-prostheses using Ceramic/Ceramic Components

M. Böhler, R. Meizer and H. Plenk

In this study the authors investigated the results of different designs of cementless THRs using ceramic/ceramic components. The authors analyzed the clinical results taking into account the age of the patients and of the type of implants used and also developed some basic considerations with regard to the interaction between Al_2O_3 ceramics and human tissue.

Clinical results obtained for 474 cementless hip endoprostheses using different designs with ceramic/ceramic components:

Materials and Methods

In the study, a number of cementless hip endoprostheses implanted beginning in 1992 utilizing a Biolox® or Biolox forte® wear couple in different design acetabular components were investigated. The group of patients involved consisted of 296 females and 178 males with the average age of the patients being 61.2 years (17 - 89 years) at the time of the operation. The patients diagnosis were: idiopathic arthrosis in 69.5% (n =329) of the patients, followed by patients with hip dysplasia (12.9 % ; n= 61) and necrosis of the femoral head (11.4%; n=54).

All of the femoral components used were made of Titanium alloy with a rectangular section and a corundum-blasted surface. The acetabular components were made of pure titanium of a either a rounded or a truncated threaded design (type A and B)(43.5%; n=206) or of a hemispherical porous coated design with either pegs or adjunctive screw fixation utilizing a press-fit technique (type C and D)(56.5%; n= 268) (Fig.1). Regardless of the type of implant utilized, the wear articulating surfaces were always either Biolox® or Biolox forte® ceramic ball heads and inserts. There were 9 special extended collar heads providing an extra long neck offset. The reason why such extralong femoral heads were used will be discussed later (see below).

Follow up was performed after a minimum interval of 2 years using the Harris Hip Score either on personal follow-up examinations or by way of telephone interviews. The x-rays which were analyzed and evaluated in accordance with the stability criteria for cementless implants of DeLee and Gruen [1,2]. Statistical analysis using the method developed by Kaplan & Meier [3] however was performed of different aspects such as age of the patients and types of prostheses used.

Type A = Screwed cup
N = 177 (37.3%)

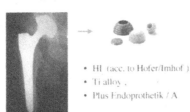

- HI (acc. to Hofer/Imhof)
- Ti alloy ,
- Plus Endoprothetik / A

Type B = Screwed cup
N = 29 (6.1%)

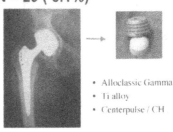

- Alloclassic Gamma
- Ti alloy
- Centerpulse / CH

Type C = Press Fit Cup
N = 230 (48.5%)

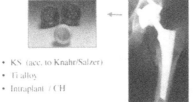

- KS (acc. to Knahr/Salzer)
- Ti alloy
- Intraplant / CH

Type D = Press Fit Cup
N = 38 (8%)

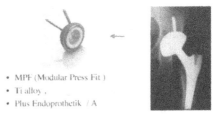

- MPF (Modular Press Fit)
- Ti alloy ,
- Plus Endoprothetik / A

Figure 1

Results

After an average follow-up period of 4 years (1 month to 15 years), 412 patients (86.9%) were re-examined. 27 patients (5.7%) had died and 35 patients (7.4%) were not available for follow up.

During the period of observation (Ø 73 months; 12 to 149 months), 12 patients were reoperated because of mechanically loosened prosthetic cups, 2 patients because of loosened stems and acetabular cups, and one patient because of a loosened stem-type prosthesis. 6 other reoperations were performed because of recurrent luxations (n=4) or deep implant infections (n=2). In 5 cases, the complications were due to fracture of the femoral head. Among these heads were 4 of 9 XL collar-type heads and 1 of 176 L heads with the latter having been implanted in combination with a small attachable adaptor. The fractures occurred after an average period of 26 months (16 – 35 months) from the date of implantation and were not caused by any adequate traumata. The average age of the patients concerned (female = 1, male = 4) was 58 years and the patients were still young and active.

An analysis of the revision data of the type of prostheses used was that 12 of the 13 prosthetic cups which were replaced were type C acetabular components (spherical press-fit cup of the Knahr & Salzer type), and one was a type A prosthesis (tapered screw cup HI). The rest of the acetabular components were found to be stable which was confirmed by the radiographs and clinical examinations. The statistical survival analysis can be seen from fig. 2 and yields a survival rate of 99.4% (type A) or 100% (types B and D) for screwed type A and B cups and for the type D press-fit cup after an average follow-up period of 18, 27 and 30 months. The survival rate for the spherical cup of the Knahr & Salzer type demonstrated a survival rate of 59.8% after an average follow-up period of 70 months.

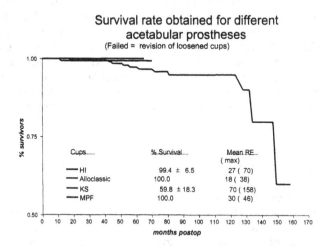

Figure 2

The results of the analysis of revisions depending on the age of the patients were divided into 3 age groups (patients < 50 years (n=62) , 51 to 65 years (n=215), > 65 years (n=197)). The revision rates were 4.8% (3 of 62) in the group of patients < 50 years; 3.2% (7 of 215) in the group of the 51 to 65 old and 1.5% (3 of 197) in the group of patients older than 65 years. Revision operations were performed after an average period of 57 months in the group of patients < 50 years, after an average period of 94 months in the group of the 51 to 65 years old, and after an average period of 72 months in the group of patients > 65 years.

Interaction between Al_2O_3 ceramics and the human tissue

In addition to the well known benefits of low abrasion and high tissue compatibility of the particles produced by the tribological system offered by the ceramic articulation of Al_2O_3 ceramics, the authors would like to point out to another important aspect which consists in the effect of the Al_2O_3 particles - i.e. of the corundum - used in the surface treatment and roughening of the titanium surfaces. Corundum is used in the production of all cementless titanium prostheses available in the market in order to provide a rougher surface for apposition to bone. Surface contamination of the implant surface by the roughening media, corundum, has been proven by scanning electron microscopy [4]. These corundum particles released from the surface invade the periprosthetic tissue at different concentration levels withsome of the smallest particles even finding their way into the articulating surfaces where they cause three-body wear. The exact migration mechanisms have not been clearly defined yet.

In addition abrasive wear of femoral heads caused by third body particles originating from hydroxy-apatite-coated porous coated stems - have already been described for prostheses systems using metal/PE component configurations [5]. Abrasive damge to the surface of metal femoral heads and metal cups caused by Al_2O_3 particles has been proven by the authors previously for prostheses using metal/metal component designs [6]. The end results of these mechanisms and their effect on wear rates can only be estimated at this point in time with the absolute extent of abrasion on both the polyethylene and the metal, we must proceed under the assumption that the periprosthetic tissues are exposed to high particle quantities under these conditions. In the case of ceramic/ceramic component configurations, the risk of three-body wear caused by mechanisms which are similar to the ones described above can be neglected because the hardness of the particles and of the prosthetic components are the same.

Conclusions

The results from the study conducted by the authors concluded that the use of Al_2O_3 ceramic components in different cementless prosthetic systems proved to be successful in all implants which followed a desing conept that provided immediate primary stability in bone to be achieved. A high number of loosened prostheses and revisions resulted from the use of one acetabular design (spherical cup of the Knahr – Salzer type) clinically. Such poor medium-term results could reasonably have been expected against the background of previous migration analyses [7]. All other implants that were followed up were found to be radiologically and clinically stable. In the investigated group of patients, there were not any resorption edges on the proximal femur or early reoperations of stable implants because of heavy pain independent of any strain conditions as have been observed recently to an increasing extent for prostheses with high-carbide and low-carbide metal/metal component configurations.

In the author's opinion, if both, the implant and the component configuration are selected correctly and if the implantation is carried out properly, the use of Al_2O_3 ceramics in cementless THR systems will provide reliable clinical results in the future in great part due to its excellent wear properties.

References

1. DeLee J., Charnley J.: (1976) Radiological demarcation of cemented sockets in total hip replacement. Clin.Orthop. 121 20-32
2. Gruen T.A., McNeice G.M., Amstutz H.C.: (1979) Modes of failure of cemented stem-type femoral components. A radiographic analysis of loosening. Clin.Orthop. 141 17-27
3. Kaplan EL,Meier (1958) P. Nonparametric estimation from incomplete observations. J Am Stat Assoc. ;53:457-81
4. A Kolb, (2002) Aluminiumoxidkeramik-Partikelrückstände auf der Oberflächenrauhigkeit von rauhgestrahlten Femurschäften [Alumina ceramic residues on the surface of coarse-blasted femoral shanks]. Dissertation a.d.Univ. Wien
5. TW Bauer et al (1996) Abrasive Three Body Wear of Polyethylene Caused by broken Filament Cables of a total hip Prosthesis. Journ Bone Joint Surg. Vol 78A,1244-7

6. M Böhler et al. (2002)Adverse tissue reactions to wear particles from Co-alloy articulations increased by alumnia blasting particle contamination from cementless Ti – blasted total hip implants. Journ Bone Joint Surg. Vol 84AB,128-36
7. Böhler M, Krismer M, Mayr G, Mühlbauer M, Salzer M : (1998)
   Migration -Measurement of cementless acetabular components Value of clinical and radiographic data Orthopedics,21,No.8,897

1.7 Alumina Ceramic against Polyethylene: A long term follow up

Ph. Hernigou, A. Nogier, A. Poignard and P. Filippini

Abstract

Between 1978 and 1990 the femoral implant was the same in four groups of patients with different function couples: alumina/alumina, (AL/AL); alumina/ polyethylene (AL/PE); metal/polyethylene (Me/PE); zirconia/polyethylene (Zir/ PE). The aim of this study was to compare survival rate, wear and femoral osteolysis among different couples of friction in patients with the same femoral stem.

For comparison between AL/AL and AL/PE we studied retrospectively 40 hips with a minimum 15 year follow-up (20 hips with an alumina/alumina (AL/AL) couple, 20 hips with an alumina/polyethylene couple (AL/PE). All the patients had the same femoral stem implanted with cement. All the cups (Al or PE) were cemented. The cause of THA was osteonecrosis for all the patients. The area of osteolysis was estimated in square millimeters on the calcar and the femur, using an image analysis program. In the alumina on alumina group the average follow-up was 18 years (range 17 to 19). Among these 20 hips, 8 cups had revision between 5 and 18 years. Among the 12 Al/Al hips without revision no osteolysis was seen before 7 years. At the most recent follow-up (average 18 years) the osteolysis is average 17 mm^2 (range 0 to 47) in these 12 hips with AL/AL couple. Among the 8 AL/AL hips with cup loosening, osteolysis before revision was average 12 mm^2 (range 0 to 32). In the AL/PE group the average follow-up is 16 years (range 15 to 17). 2 PE cups had revision at 12 and 13 years. In the 18 AL/PE hips without revision osteolysis was average 106 mm^2 at 15 years (range 31 to 254 mm^2). In the 2 Al/PE hips with cup loosening osteolysis was 215 and 310 mm^2 before revision. Even with cup loosening, osteolysis was lower in the AL/AL group.

For comparison between AL/PE and Zir/PE we studied hips with the two different ceramics during the same period and with a minimum ten year follow-up. All the patients had the same stem implanted with cement. The polyethylene of the cemented cup was the same. The femoral head was made of dense alumina (Al$_2$O$_3$) with a diameter of 32 mm in sixty-two cases and made of yttrium-oxide-partially-stabilized zirconia with a diameter of 28 mm in forty cases. These hips were compared with a Me/PE group. No osteolysis of the calcar was seen before three years; at the fifth year of follow-up, the osteolysis was similar in the two groups. At the lastest follow-up (twelve years), the average wear rate of the alumina group was 0.07 mm/year during the last year; in the zirconia group an increase of the wear rate was observed between the 5th and the 12th year. In the zirconia group the average wear rate was 0.4 mm/year at the twelve year follow-up. The osteolysis was greater in the zirconia group (average 255 mm^2) than in the alumina group (average 35 mm^2) at the lastest follow-up. The total amount of wear at the most recent follow-up was average 1360 cubic millimeters for the zirconia group and 755 cubic millimeters for the alumina group. In the Me/PE group wear and osteolysis were higher than in the AL/PE group.

On long term follow up, the AL/AL had less osteolysis than the other couples of friction. However the survivorship was better for the AL/PE than for the AL/AL in the very long term (between 15 and 20 years follow up). Zir/PE and metal/PE had increased osteolysis and lower survivorship than AL/PE.

References:

1. Hernigou P., Nogier A.: Femoral osteolysis in hips with alumina/alumina in comparison with alumina against PE. AAOS; mars 2001.
2. Hernigou P., Bahrami T.: Zirconia and alumina ceramics in comparison with stainless-steel heads. J. Bone Joint Surg. Br 2003; 85-B: 504-509.

SESSION 2

Advanced Ceramic Applications
and New Projects

2.1 Long Term Wear of Ceramic on Ceramic Hips

J. Fisher, J. Nevelos, T. D. Stewart, J. L. Tipper and E. Ingham

First and second generation alumina on alumina bearings in hip prostheses showed low long term wear rates in vivo 1 mm³/year with a characteristic style wear pattern on the head, thought to be associated with cup rim contact [1]. Standard laboratory simulator studies have failed to replicate this wear rate or mechanism [2,3]. In 1999 we developed a new hip simulation method which replicates joint laxity, microseparation and head cup rim contact [4], and this has been show to replicate wear rates, mechanism and debris found in third generation hip and alumina on alumina Biolox Forte bearings [4,5,6,7,8]. The wear rates of these third generation bearings is at least ten fold less than highly cross linked polyethylene. Additionally, the ceramic wear debris has been found to be less reactive than cross linked polyethylene [9,10] resulting in substantially lower functional osteolytic potential. Using these novel simulator methods fourth generation Biolox Delta alumina matrix components, have shown further reduction in wear compared to third generation Biolox Forte bearings [11].

References

1. Nevelos JE, Ingham E, Doyle C, Nevelos AB, Fisher J. Analysis of retrieved alumina ceramic components for Mittelmeier total hip prostheses. Biomaterials, 20, 1833-1840 (1999).
2. Nevelos JE, Ingham E, Doyle C, Nevelos AB, Fisher J. The influence of acetabular cup angle on the wear of "BIOLOX Forte" alumina ceramic bearing couples in a hip joint simulator. Journal of Materials Science: Materials in Medicine 12, 141-144 (2001).
3. Nevelos JE, Ingham E, Doyle C, Nevelos AB, Fisher J. Wear of HIPed and non-HIPed alumina-alumina hip joints under standard and severe simulator testing conditions. Jnl of Biomaterials 22, 2191-2197 (2001).
4. Nevelos J, Ingham E, Doyle C, Streicher R, Nevelos A, Walter W, Fisher J. Microseparation of the centers of alumina-alumna artificial hip joints during simulator testing produces clinically relevant wear and patterns. The Journal of Arthroplasty 15, 793-795 (2000).
5. Nevelos JE, Prudhommeaux, Hamadouche M, Doyle C, Ingham E, Meunier A, Nevelos AB, Sedel L, Fisher J. Comparative analysis of two different types of alumina-alumina hip prosthesis retrieved for aseptic loosening. Jnl of Bone and Joint Surgery, Vol. 83-B, No. 4, 598-603 (2001).
6. Tipper JL, Firkins PJ, Besong AA, Barbour PSM, Nevelos J, Stone MH, Ingham E, Fisher J. Characterisation of wear debris from UHMWPE on zirconia ceramic, metal-on-metal and alumina ceramic-on-ceramic hip prostheses generated in a physiological anatomical hip joint simulator. Wear 250, 120-128, 2001.
7. Hatton A, Nevelos JE, Nevelos AA, Banks RE, Fisher J, Ingham E. Alumina-alumina artificial hip joints. Part I: A histological analysis and characterisation of wear debris by laser capture microdissection of tissues retrieved at revision. Biomaterials 23, 3429-3440 (2002).
8. Tipper JL, Hatton A, Nevelos JE, Ingham E, Doyle C, Streicher R, Nevelos AB, Fisher J. Alumina-alumina artificial hip joints. Part II: Characterisation of the wear debris from in vitro hip joints simulations. Biomaterials 23, 3441-3448 (2002).

9. Hatton A, Nevelos JE, Matthew JB, Fisher J, Ingham E. Effects of clinically relevant alumina ceramic wear particles on TNF-* production by human peripheral blood mononuclear phagocytes. Biomaterials 24, 1193-1204 (2003).
10. Fisher J, Ingham E, Stone MH. Alternative bearing couples in total hip replacements: Solutions for young patients HIP International Vol 13 31-35 (2003).
11. Stewart TD, Tipper JL, Insley G, Streicher RM, Ingham E, Fisher J. Long-term wear of ceramic matrix composite materials for hip prostheses under severe swing phase microseparation. Journal of Biomedical Materials Research, Applied Biomaterials, Part B, 66B, 567-573, 2003.

2.2 Periarticular Reaction to Wear Debris of Different Ceramic Materials

G. Maccauro, C. Piconi, F. Muratori, S. Sangiorgi, A. Sgambato, W. Burger, P. Dalla Pria, M. Esposito and A. Cittadini

Introduction

For the last 30 years Alumina and Zirconia ceramics constituted the ceramic materials used for the manufacturing of Total Joint Arthroplasty, thanks to the high biological and mechanical properties of these materials (Piconi and al, 2003; Piconi and Maccauro 1999). The new ceramic biocomposite ZPTA (Alumina Matrix Composites by Transformation Toughened and in situ Plateled Reinforcement) that is currently known as Biolox® delta, produced by CeramTec (namely ZPTA in the paper), improving the mechanical properties when compared to Alumina (Burger W. and Richter H.G. 2000), allowed to manufacture components which were not previously possible, and especially the small-diameter ball heads (<28 mm), thin-walled cup insert, knee and finger joints. Few paper reported the in vitro and in vivo biocompatibility tests on this new material (Willmann, et al. 2000), and in particular as ceramic joints are intended for use in younger patient (Black 1997, Schmalzried 2001), hence the ones with longer life expectations, the study of the chronic effects of small particles, in term of local and systemic toxicity, including carcinogenesys becomes more and more relevant (Archimbeck et al. 2000).

In a previous paper (Maccauro et al., 2002) we described an in vivo test suitable for the observation of biological reactions made in an animal model of chronic release of ceramic particles with the observations made in case of release of ceramic particles from THR joints due to wear or fracture.

The in-vivo model of particle release that we used is based on the implant of porous pellets formed by low cohesion grains in the patellar tendon of rabbits. Due to their poor cohesion, when rubbing against an articular cartilage, grains can be easily and progressively detached from the surface of the pellet and released to the joint space all along the nursing time of the animals. In this paper we would like to present the first results obtained, compared the biological response to Alumina, Zirconia and ZPTA ceramics).

Materials and Methods

Ceramic pellets (Ø 8 x 2 mm) were manufactured from Alumina, Yttria Tetragonal Zirconia Policrystals (Y-TZP in this paper) and ZPTA precursors by cold pressing followed by pressure less sintering route. The results were compared with the ones obtained by the insertion of the ceramic precursors in form of powders in the articular joint.

Pellets are characterised by high porosity obtained stopping the sintering process during the development phase of the necks between the grains of the starting powder. Thanks to this system, the cohesion among grains in the pellets is very low.

Twenty four New Zealand White adult rabbits of both sex, minimum weight 3.3 Kg were used for the experiments and divided in 3 groups. The pellets of each ceramic were inserted into surgically created defects under both the patellar tendons of 8 rabbits for the first group. Animals were maintained in a pathogen-free environment.

At different intervals (1, 3, 6, 12 months after surgery) the animals were killed. Knee joints were harvested and submitted to macroscopic and x-rays examinations. Retrieved knees were divided in 2 groups: specimens of the first group were decalcified with EDTA, dehydrated and embedded in paraffin, sectioned and stained with hematoxylin-eosin, and observed with transmitted and polarised light microscopy. Pellets of the second group were removed, fixed in Karnosky's solution dehydrated with alcohol, and examined by SEM (Philips 515).

Two animals of each group (Alumina, Y-TZP and ZPTA) for each implantation time, was submitted to autopsy. Lungs, liver, kidney, spleen and hearth were harvested, and the external and internal surfaces of these organs underwent macroscopic examinations. Lungs were injected with China ink for detecting tumours. Histological analysis was carried out on specimens of the organs fixed in 10% formalin, embedded in paraffin, cut in 3-5 μm thin sections, stained with haematoxylin-eosin and resorcin-fuchsin.

Results

The preliminary results of the study are reported in this paper: in particular the in vivo results at 1 month after operation of the 3 groups.

Macroscopic analysis of the retrieved rabbit knees showed the presence of fibrosis around the joint at 1 month after operation, independently on the materials tested, fixing in flexion the knees. X-ray showed the presence of ceramic fragments in the articular spaces, with Alumina and Y-TPZ pellets, but not in case of ZPTA. Histologic sections in case of Alumina showed ceramic particles within histiocyte-like cells as finely dispersed intracytoplasmatic granules or as yellow-brown bigger granules in extracellular matrix of a synovial-like tissue. Giant cells containing bigger ceramic fragments were rarely seen. Y-TZP grains appeared or as dark structure in the intercellular space, or as microscopic yellow amber grains found in intra or in extra cellular sites, scattered in areas of cell reaction containing mononuclear histiocyte-like cells. Membranes were characterised by avascular fibrous tissue. In case of ZPTA a tissue membrane containing multinuclear cells surrounded the retrieved pellets. Granules were not visible at histology. The peripheral organs did not show pathological changes neither tumours. SEM of the membranes surrounding pellets showed the presence of ceramic grains: in case of Alumina particles appeared as alone or aggregate due to electrostatic reactions, in case of Y-TZP and in case of ZPTA particles were usually alone (average Ø 2 μm).

Discussion

It is well known that wear is the key factor to artroprostheses' lifetime: at local level the cascade of events induced by reactions to wear debris is still the most frequent cause of implant failure and revision, while the ions released by wear debris originate systemic reactions, depending on their transport by the blood flow to peripheral organs, thanks to the vascularization of the reactive membrane surrounding the implant. (Schmalzried and Callaghan 1999, Urban et al. 2000, Archimbeck et al. 2000, Fisher et al 2001, Sedel 2001, Dumbleton et al. 2002). The biocompatibility tests for a candidate biomaterial for Orthopaedic implants should similar the biological events which take place in presence of biomaterial or its wear products.

The in vivo tests used to evaluate tissue reactions to particulate materials analyze the biological response to the particle directly injected in the joint (Rae et al 1986), or in packing the powders on a suitable carrier, like e.g. into the groove in a PMMA cylinder, and in implanting the carrier into the joint (Kubo et al 1999). These methods have some limits: particles injection is similar to the clinical situation of massive release of particles in case of catastrophic failure of the implant, but is different from the usual clinical situation of chronic release of wear debris, that is low in case of metals and very low in case of ceramics; the use of PMMA as carrier may influence the results obtained due the contamination of different materials.

Moreover in case of ceramic materials the in vivo tests should evaluate the chronic effects of the materials in order to predict if the material tested may really be used in younger patients, that will make use of the implant for longer times (e.g. thirty years, or more).

The method used analyzed the local and systemic effects to Alumina, Y-TZP and ZPTA ceramics. Each pellets consisted of only one material without contaminations of cement or any other carrier. The entity of cohesion is crucial in the effects as well as the animal joint motion: we observe more particles at 1 month after operation released from Alumina and Y-TZP than from ZPTA, either at XRay either histology, and only with SEM we observed the presence of ceramic particles in the periprosthetic tissue.

The reaction to the Alumina an Y-TZP ceramic particles in the articular joints was the formation of fibrous tissue, characterized by the absence of blood vessels, and by a cellular reaction depending on the size of the particles released. We observed in our specimens the presence of few giant cells, clearly related to ceramics only. In case of ZPTA ceramics multinuclear cells were present in the periprosthetic membrane: no vessels were seen in the tissue.

The membranes were poor in vessels in case of Alumina and Y-TZP and no vessels were seen in presence of delta at 1 month after operation, showing that materials do not induce an inflammatory reaction similar to the one induced by metals (Willert et al. 1996). We remark that lymphatic vessels collect particles and transport materials to the peripheral organs, and is related to a possible systemic toxicity of materials: the absence of vessels as observed in case of ZPTA may be an indirect sign of low toxicity and of systemic safety in case of implantation in younger patients. No tissue damages were seen in the peripheral organs whatever materials were used, no tumours were seen in the animals.

Obviously more information should be kept from the long term results for confirming the suitability of the materials, and the absence of cancer risk of these ceramics.

Conclusions

We conclude that the method proposed may be considered a useful system for evaluating the chronic effects of ceramic materials, thanks to the friction of low cohesive materials against cartilage and release of low entity of wear debris, comparable to the in vivo situation of well performing prostheses, implanted in younger patients with a longer expectation.

At 1 month after operation we did not observe local or systemic toxicity due to material tested, neither tumours developed.

A poor in vessels membrane surrounds Alumina and Y-TZP pellets, revealing the lack of inflammatory reaction to these materials, with a possible transport of debris released to the peripheral organs; in particular the absence of vessels observed in the tissue membranes surrounding ZPTA seems to reveal that this material is especially indicated in younger patients.

References

1. Archibeck MJ, Jacobs JJ, Black J (2000) Alternate bearing surfaces in total joint arthroplasty: biologic considerations. Clin Orthop 379:12-21

2. Black J (1997) Prospects for alternate Bearing surfaces in total hip replacement arthroplasty of the hip. In: Puhl W (ed) Performance of the wear couple BIOLOX Forte in hip arthroplasty, Enke Verlag, Stuttgart, pp 2-10

3. Burger W, Richter HG (2000) High Strength and Toughness Alumina Matrix Composites by Transformation Toughened and in situ Plateled Reinforcement (ZPTA) – The New Generation of Bioceramics. Bioceramics 13: 545-548.

4. Dumbleton JH, Manley MT, Edidin AA (2002) A literature review of the association between wear rate and osteolysis in total hip arthroplasty. J Arthroplasty 17:649-661

5. Fisher J, Stone MH, Tipper JL, Ingham E. (2001) Wear debris generation with metal-on-polyethylene, Metal-on Metal, Ceramic-on-Ceramic hip prostheses. In: Rieker C, Oberholzer S, Wyss U (eds) World Tribology Forum in Arthroplasty. Hans Huber, Bern, pp 25-30

6. Kubo T, Sawada K, Hirakava K, et al (1999) Histiocite reaction in rabbit femurs to UHMWPE, metal, and ceramic particles in different sizes. J Biomed Mater Res 45:363-369

7. Maccauro G, Piconi C, Muratori F, De Santis V, Burger W (2002) Tissue reactions to ceramic wear debris: clinical cases vs animal model (Proc. 8th BIOLOX Symp. Bioceramics in joint Arthroplasty, Zippel H and Dietrich M Eds) 81-87

8. Piconi C., Maccauro G., Muratori F., Brach del Prever E. (2003) Alumina and zirconia ceramics in joint replacements J. Applied Biomaterials & Biomechanics 1:19-32.

9. Piconi C. and Maccauro G. (1999) Zirconia as a ceramic biomaterial. Biomaterials 20:1-25

10. Rae T (1986) The macrophage to implant materials with special reference to those used in Orthopaedics. CRC Crit Rev Biocomp 2: 97

11. Schmalzried TP, Callaghan JJ (1999) Current Concepts Review: Wear in total hip and knee replacements. J Bone Joint Surg 81-A:115-136

12. Schmalzried TP (2001) Patient activity and wear. In: Rieker C, Oberholzer S, Wyss U (eds) World Tribology Forum in Arthroplasty. Hans Huber, Bern, 31-34

13. Sedel L (2001) Tribology of hip joint replacement. In: Surgical techniques in Orthopedics and Traumatology, Edition Scientifiques et Medicales Elsevier SAS, Paris, 55-430-E-10

14. Urban RM, Jacobs JJ, Tomlinson MJ, et al (2000) Dissemination of wear particles to the liver, spleen, and abdominal lymph nodes of patients with hip or knee replacement. J Bone Joint Surg 82-A: 457-477

15. Willert MG, Broback LG, Buchan GM, et al (1996) Crevice corrosion of cemented titanium alloy stems in total hip replacement. Clin Ortop 333:51-75

16. Willmann G, von Chamier W, Pfaff HG, Rock R (2000) Biocompatibility of a New Alumina Matrix Biocomposite AMG Bioceramics 13 :569-572

2.3 Two Bearing Ceramic Surfaces with a Self Adjusting Cup: A New Solution to avoid Dislocation and Subluxation in Total Hip Prosthesis

J.-Y. Lazennec, Chen Qingshan, An Kai Nan and B. Masson

Introduction

Dislocation remains one of the most common complications after total hip arthroplasty.

The ceramic on ceramic bearing surface hasn't yet solved this problem.

Its prevalence ranges from 0.6% to 7% according to different publications series. [1-2-3-4-5-6-7-8-9]. These wide variations are related to the type of hip surgery, the type of prosthesis used, the patient's characteristics, surgical techniques, and the surgeon's experience.

Ceramic on ceramic requires a more exacting technique and component position. Intra operative assessment is more critical [10]. Dislocation is a major cause of failure of Ce-Ce prosthesis compared to a classical Metal PE bearing couple (0,51% versus 0,14%). [11].

Precise cup position appears to be a main factor influencing the risk of dislocation.

Clinical studies show that the dislocation risk is 6,9 times higher if total anteversion is not between 40° and 60° after THA [12]. This accentuates the interest in alternatives with 3D. Ceramic Self Adjusting Cup joint as anteversion variations also occurs according to sitting or standing positions. [13-14].

Anatomical and geometrical study

Three dimensional analysis of dislocation and micro separation demonstrates that some factors are related to prosthesis design and surgical implantation. But one of the main problems remains the lack of accuracy in pre and per-operative planification, mainly for the acetabular cup: different morphological and functional parameters depending on the patient are more or less controlled during surgical implantation:

1. The range of motion of a normal spine induces variation of sagittal acetabular tilt between standing and sitting position. The modifications of sagittal orientation are associated with less cup anteversion in standing position and more cup anteversion in sitting position.

2. Diseases affecting lumbosacral junction and/or prior surgical procedures (ageing spine, lumbosacral fusion) reduce the adaptation of T.H.P. to sitting or standing position.

   In patients with limited spinal motion and/or permanent backward rotation of the pelvis, changes in anteversion between the sitting and standing position may be very small. This explains the possible catastrophic consequences of selecting an inappropriate position during hip replacement.

3. Regarding those morphological and functional parameters, acetabular implantation is an arbitrary compromise. Standardising the position of the patient and the operative technique does not eliminate the risk of sub optimal acetabular cup positioning in patients with unusual anatomical characteristics.

Furthermore hip prosthesis articulations currently used are non anatomical, and therefore don't have the mechanical characteristics and tolerance of the natural hip.

3D▲ Ceramic Self Adjusting Cup solution.

The use of 3D▲ ceramic self adjusting cup joint seems an interesting alternative to face those difficult situations for adjustment and hip stability as, in some cases, no ideal solution can be found for acetabular implantation.

One manner of increasing the stability of an artificial joint is to modify the position of the rotation centre. Some publications explain that an inset of few millimetres increases the peak resisting moment. [15-16]. The moment necessary applied to get dislocation must be higher. This benefit in term of stability has a big disadvantage in loss of range of motion.

The 3D▲ system has allowed to move the rotation centre much deeper inside the insert without any impact on the ROM, in other terms the 3D Delta could give more stability with a comparable ROM as a standard system.

A study in collaboration with the CEA (Atomic Research Centre) explains in detail the behaviour of these 3 ceramics components. The "Self adaptation" of the intermediate cup can be demonstrated: the additional outer-bearing surface motion creates a second "adjustable acetabulum"

After defining different parameters (Inclination of the insert 45°, Forces and Moment applied on rotation centre) a comparison of the mechanism of dislocation between a standard system (composed of a Ball head against an Insert) and the 3D▲ system (composed of two ceramic on ceramic bearing surfaces with a self adjusting cup) has been performed.

With the Standard system, the dislocation appears if a contact occurs between the neck and the insert because of the moment applied. This dislocation by impingement is in direct relation with the range of motion.

With the 3D▲ system, the mechanism is different and shows different steps:

- Rotation of the Ball head alone.
- Rotation of the Bipolar head in the opposite direction because of contact forces, until contact between the Bipolar head and the stem.
- Finally rotation of the Ball head and the Bipolar head will appear together.

This Self adjusting cup phenomena is now well described and due to the eccentration of the Bipolar head from the Ball head; the phenomena is different to the workings of a classical tripolar prosthesis.

With "h" the offset between the rotation centre of the ball head and the rotation centre of the bipolar head, applied forces are not on the same application point. This offset creates a resultant force Fr that rotates the bipolar head until its adjustment .

Two Biomechanical studies in the USA and in Europe are ongoing and will confirm the resistance to dislocation of the 3D▲ system, compared to other systems available on the market.

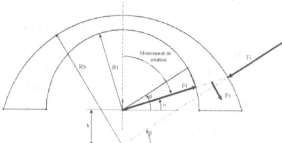

Figure 1:
Self Adjusting Cup Mechanism.

Mechanical performance

In collaboration with CeramTec AG a qualification program has been established to evaluate the mechanical reliability of this device.
The system is made by 3 ceramics components:

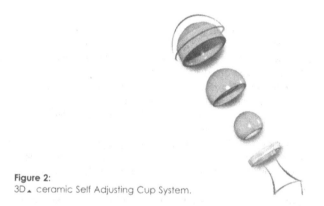

Figure 2:
3D ceramic Self Adjusting Cup System.

A standard ball head of 22,2 mm, a Bipolar head (intermediate piece) and a standard XLW fix insert 32/41 mm.
A standard qualification program for the Ball Head and the fix insert has been performed. Concerning the Bipolar head, a new program has been set up based on a ball head qualification program. Specifications of the Bipolar head, diameter, roundness, clearance, etc... are strictly the same as a 32mm ceramic ball head.
All 3 components have successfully passed the qualification. Mechanical characteristics of Biolox® Delta enable the manufacturing of this special device and especially of the intermediate cup with excellent strength properties.
Finally, tests have been performed to evaluate the resistance of the PE ring to secure the ball head inside the intermediate piece. Results are comparable to similar PE rings used for more than 18 years with double mobility Metal Polyethylene.
Previous tribological tests with Biolox® Delta bearing couples show very low wear rate.
Currently a study is on going in the Bio-mechanical Laboratory in Leeds (UK) over 20 Mc on standard hip simulator and on Hip simulator with microseparation.

Conclusion

3D▲ self adjusting cup joint offers new solutions to reduce the risk of dislocation and sub luxation. The device also reduces the wear by using the new ceramic Biolox® delta.

The decision to use the 3D▲ device could be made preoperatively. The surgeon could decide during the operation if the patient needs a classical Ceramic on Ceramic bearing couple or the 3D▲ system in case of concerns about stability. The device could also be used against a PE insert to have a benefit in stability only.

Reducing the risk of dislocation and reducing drastically wear are two advantages that could place the 3D▲ system as the best choice in primary Total Hip Arthroplasty. Obviously this choice applies to recurrent dislocation also.

The use of the 3D▲ device could have a positive impact in terms of cost by reducing significantly the number of revisions.

References

1. Lewinnek GE, Lewis JL, Tarr R, Compere CL, Zimmerman JR. Dislocation after total hip replacement arthroplasties. Journal of Bone and Joint Surgery, 60, 1978: 217-220.
2. Fackler CD, Poss R. Dislocation in total hip arthroplasties. Clinical Orthopaedics and Related Research, 1980: 169-178.
3. Ali Khan MA, Brakenbury PH, Reynolds IS. Dislocation following total hip replacement. Journal of Bone and Joint Surgery-British Volume, 63-B, 1981: 214-218.
4. Woo RY, Morrey BF. Dislocations after total hip arethroplasty. Journal of Bone and Joint Surgery, 64, 1982: 1295-1306.
5. Kavanagh BF, Fitzgerald RH, Jr. Multiple revisions for failed total hip arthroplasty not associated with infection. Journal of Bone and Joint Surgery, 69, 1987: 1144-1149.
6. Morrey BF. Instability after total hip arthroplasty. Orthopedic Clinics of North America, 23, 1992: 237-248.
7. Berry DJ. Unstable total hip arthroplasty: detailed overview. Instructional Courses Lecture, 50, 2001: 265-274.
8. Sanchez-Sotelo J, Berry DJ. Epidemiology of instability after total hip replacement. Orthopedic Clinics of North America, 32, 2001: 543-552.
9. Von Knoch M. Berry DJ. Harmsen WS. Morrey BF. Late dislocation after total hip arthroplasty. Journal of Bone & Joint Surgery - American Volume. 84-A(11):1949-53, 2002
10. William J. Maloney USA Current Concept Joint Replacement Spring 03 Las Vegas .
11. Toni, A. Sudanese Bioceramics in joint arthroplasty Ed Thieme March 2001 Ceramic on ceramic: Long term clinical experience
12. Jolles BM, Zangger P, Leyvraz PF. Factors predisposing to dislocation after primary total hip arthroplasty: a multivariate analysis. Journal of Arthroplasty,17, 2002: 282-288.
13. Lazennec JY, Charlot N, Gorin M, Roger B, Arafati N, Bissery A, Saillant G. Hip-spine relationship: a radio-anatomical study for optimization in acetabular cup positioning. Surgical & Radiologic Anatomy. 25(7), 2003
14. Eddine TA. Migaud H. Chantelot C. Cotten A. Fontaine C. Duquennoy A. Variations of pelvic anteversion in the lying and standing positions: analysis of 24 control subjects and implications for CT measurement of position of a prosthetic cup. Surgical & Radiologic Anatomy. 23(2): 105-10, 2001

15. Scifert CF, Brown TD, Pedersen DR, Callaghan JJ. A finite element analysis of factors influencing total hip dislocation. Clinical Orthopaedics and Related Research, 1998: 152-162.
16. Scifert CF, Brown TD, Lipman JD. Finite element analysis of a novel design approach to resisting total hip dislocation. Clinical Biomechanics 1999: 697-703.

2.4 Analysis and Investigation of the Adhesive Strength of Ceramic and Bone Cement in Knee Arthroplasty

S. Leyen, S. Vetter and H. Plank

Introduction

Ceramic total knee arthroplasty is not popular at present. Though good experiences of total hip replacement showed that ceramic-ceramic coupling proved itself as a long-time implant. Knee endoprosthesis should be fixed in place with bone cement. The implant-cement interface affects significantly the mechanical situation of the total system and can cause loosening of the implant. As loosening of the implant is one of the most common reasons for failure of the prosthesis, measurements of the strength of these bonds are of great interest.

Purpose

This study is attending to find practical ways for strengthening ceramic / bone cement interface via mechanical and chemical surface treatment. Furthermore the thickness of the cement layer as well as an immersion in moisture environment was tested on adhesive strength of the ceramic-cement interface. In addition, the adhesive strength of ceramic / bone cement interface and the coupling of TiAl6V4 / bone cement was compared.

Method

To determine the adhesive strength of ceramic / cement through tensile tests on an universal testing machine (Instron 8561 with gimbal suspension), wafers of zirconiumdioxid- and platelet reinforced aluminumoxide-ceramic (BIOLOX® delta, CeramTec AG) were bonded to metal stamps and coupled by bone cement (Palamed® G, Biomet-Merck).

Several surface structures (grooves, drills) and surface roughness created by sandblasting and polishing were applied to the ceramic surface.

To gain a chemical coupling between bone cement to ceramic some specimens were conditioned by silanisation and by an additional silicatisation.

In order to examine the hydrolytic resistance of the ceramic-cement compound the specimens were immersed for 30, 60 and 80 days in physiological saline solution at 37°C.

The adhesive strength of TiAl6V4 / cement was tested with smooth and sand-blasted surface.

Five specimens for each condition were tested to ensure a representative average value.

Results

The examination of the thickness of the cement layer showed that with thinner cement layer an enhancement of tensile bond strength can be determined. Untreated test bodies with a cement layer of 2 mm reached a tensile bond strength of 6,17 MPa (SD: ±1,38 MPa), whereas with a thinner cement layer of 0,7 mm the tensile bond strength increased to 14,90 MPa (SD: ±2,54 MPa). The reasons are more shrinkage stress and inhomogenety in thicker cement layers, which results in a lower tensile bond strength (Fig.1).

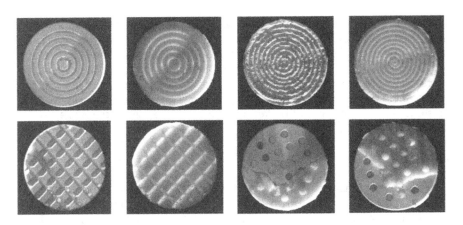

Figure 1:
Delaminating of structured samples BIOLOX® delta / Palamed® G.

Because of formation of a chemical bonding between ceramic and bone cement by silanisation the tensile bond strength stepped up significantly (Fig.2).

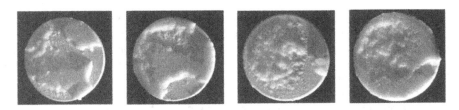

Figure 2:
Delaminating of chemical activated samples BIOLOX® delta / Palamed® G.

The increase of the adhesive strength by silanisation showed best results using polished specimens with the lowest surface roughness. Silanisation strengthens only specific adherence, because mechanical adherence on a smooth surface is marginal.

Silanisation improved tensile bond strength of the polished specimens to 135%, whereby the increase at untreated specimens was 70% and at sandblasted specimens 10%.

An additional silicatisation before silanisation could increase the tensile bond strength again, as the silane adhesion primer can build a stronger bonding to SiO_2- than to Al_2O_3-particles. The ratio of untreated to silane-conditioned to silane-conditioned and silicated specimens was 1 : 1,7 : 2.

Specimens with surface structures (grooves and drills) reduced the tensile bond strength to 10-40%. In comparison to untreated specimens. An increase of the tensile bond strength to 70% could be achieved by sandblasting, as thereby mechanical adherence could be enlarged by creating undercuts. But sandblasting is not the best for ceramic components, because it can possible damage the components.

The comparison to TiAl6V4 showed that their tensile bond strength is only 17% above the tensile bond strength of ceramic.

After immersion for 30 days in physiological saline solution at 37°C untreated specimens had an decrease of tensile bond strength of 90%, after 60 days they lost their adhesive strength completely (Fig. 3).

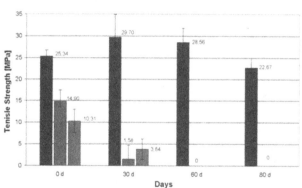

Figure 3:
Tensile strength of BIOLOX® delta / Palamed® G activated und non activated samples after 30, 60 and 80 days in Ringer solution at 37°C, Cement layer: 0,7mm.

Specimens with grooves had an decrease of tensile bond strength of 60% after immersed for 30 days. Because of fewer capillary forces in the grooves the decrease of adhesive strength is lower than at untreated specimens. Supposably specimens with grooves will also loose their adhesive strength completely after immersion for a longer period of time.

Silane-conditioned specimens showed a nearly unchanged mechanical stability after immersed for 80 days. The chemical bonding created by silanisation prevented penetration of the saline solution.

Conclusions

Recapitulating a silanisation can improve the adhesive strength between ceramic and bone cement, which is also hydrolytic resistant after immersion in physiological saline solution for 80 days. An additional silicatisation can enhance the adhesive strength again. As thinner cement layers can increase the tensile bond strength, the cement pockets in femur- and tibia-components should not be too deep.

2.5 Alumina Ceramic-Ceramic Total Hip Arthroplasty using Computer-Assisted Surgical Navigation and a New Minimally Invasive Technique

S.B. Murphy

Introduction

Proper component positioning, preservation of the soft tissue surrounding the hip, and minimization of wear are three critical components for optimizing outcome following total hip arthroplasty. The current manuscript describes methods of ensuring proper component positioning using surgical navigation and a new tissue preserving minimally invasive surgical technique, both used in combination with alumina ceramic-ceramic total hip arthroplasty.

Improper component positioning has been shown to increase the incidence of dislocation following total hip arthroplasty and to increase the rate of wear and wear induced osteolysis. Proper acetabular component positioning is especially challenging because pelvic position is not accurately known during surgery and pelvic position changes significantly during surgery. Further, intraoperative radiographs are often deceiving since these views are rarely truly antero-posterior with significant malrotation about the longitudinal and transverse axes.

Surgical navigation offers the ability to track component position accurately with system accuracies within 1mm and 1 degree. While image-free hip navigation based on percutaneously digitized landmarks can be unreliable, with large and unquantifiable errors potentially introduced at surgery, surgical navigation based on CT or intraoperative fluoroscopic images can be very efficient and accurate, adding very little time, if any, to the surgery and ensuring that components are placed in acceptable position (DiGioia, Murphy).

While at first glance, less invasive techniques, may only offer short term, but no long term benefit, the principle of preserving all of the important structures around the hip joint is well founded. The principle of tissue preservation may facilitate early recovery because these methods are also minimally invasive, but the greatest benefit may be in the long term for hip joint stability, muscle strength, and the more normal state of the soft tissues surrounding the joint at the time of any revision procedure.

The use of alumina ceramic-ceramic bearings is similarly logical and appropriate. Wear debris and debris-associated osteolysis are the most common problems affecting total hip arthroplasty. Of the three types of bearings developed to reduce wear, alumina ceramic-ceramic bearings have the greatest scientific and clinical support. The other two methods include metal-metal bearings and metal-cross linked polyethylene bearings. Ironically, while cross linked polyethylene is used most commonly, it has the shortest clinical experience (only since 1998) and the highest wear. Preliminary studies have shown measureable and only slightly improved wear (Digas). One prospective study has shown a modest (50%) reduction in wear (Martell) whereas hard bearings have shown wear reduction of more than 1,000 fold. These bearings are also still susceptible to scratching and third body debris (Endo, Fischer) and clinical examples of osteolysis have been reported for both electron beam (Reis) and gamma irradiated polyethylene bearings.

By contrast, alumina ceramic bearings have been in clinical use for more than 20 years and clinical retrievals have show linear wear rates that are 4,000X less than metal-on-polyethylene bearings of the same era (Dorlot). These bearings have consistently shown low wear rates in laboratory evaluations as well as clinically (Bizot, Boutin, Garino, Murphy). Hamadouche et al had no cases of osteolysis in un-cemented ceramic-ceramic THA's at minimum 18.5-year follow up (Hamadouche).

This current manuscript reports on the results of a prospective study of alumina-alumina bearings in total hip arthroplasty, a subset of these arthroplasties performed with computer-assisted surgical navigation, and a subset performed with both tissue-preserving, minimally-invasive techniques combined with surgical navigation.

Materials and Methods

261 total hip arthroplasties in 237 patients were performed by a single surgeon using an alumina ceramic-ceramic bearing (Wright Medical Technology, Arlington, TN and Biolox Forte XLW acetablular liners and femoral heads by Ceramtec AG, Plochingen, Germany, Figure 1). Of these, 148 were performed using computer-assisted surgical navigation and 72 were performed using a combination of computer assistance and a tissue-preserving, minimally invasive technique.

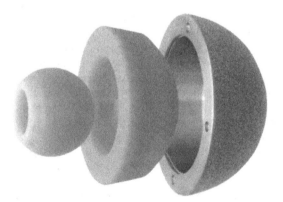

Figure 1:
The alumina-alumina bearing (Wright Medical Technology, Memphis, TN and Ceramtec AG, Plochingen, Germany).

Overall, there were 128 left hips and 133 right hips. 143 were performed in men and 108 were performed in women. Mean patient age at surgery was 50.7 years (Range: 17 years – 74 years). Patients operated upon prior to February 3, 2003 were part of an FDA/IDE study. The protocol called for patients to be evaluated clinically and radiographically twice in the first year and annually thereafter.

148 of these procedures were performed with surgical navigation either based on preoperative CT imaging (BrainLAB, Germany) or intraoperative fluoroscopy. No procedures were performed using imageless navigation since accuracy cannot be assured intra-operatively with imageless hip navigation methods. Of these 148 procedures, 72 were performed using fully tissue-preserving surgical techniques.

Design of Tissue Preserving Total Hip Arthroplasty Techniques

Design of any minimally invasive total hip technique requires decisions regarding patient position, dependence on or independence from imaging and or traction, the ability to perform a trial reduction, and the tissue intervals to be used to avoid releasing important structures.

Patient Position: The lateral position was chosen for several reasons. With the lateral position, gravity facilitates separation of the subcutaneous tissue layers and the posterior borders of the gluteus medius and medius are easily visualized. Further, this position is the most common position THA used in the United States and so surgeons who adopt this method will be able to transition the surgery into a familiar, conventional technique if any aspect of the surgery cannot be adequately managed through a more limited tissue interval.

Tissue Intervals: Since the gluteus medius, gluteus minimus, psoas, tensor fascia femoris, and rectus femoris muscles and posterior capsule are critical to hip joint function and stability, any tissue preserving surgical technique for THA must be performed without disturbing these structures. Specifically, components must be inserted either posterior, anterior, or inferior to the gluteus medius and minimus. Splitting or releasing the origin or insertion of the gluteus medius or gluteus minimus is not tissue preserving by definintion. Similarly, the posterior capsule is so essential to hip joint stability that posteriorly-based exposures involving release and repair of these structures are not tissue preserving, no matter how small the incision. Further, posterior displacement of the femoral head out of the acetabulum requires such disruption of these structures, that the femoral head cannot be posteriorly dislocated during surgery, but rather, must be either excised or dislocated anteriorly.

Anterior exposures such as the Watson-Jones and the Smith-Petersen exposures provide excellent visualization of the acetabulum but poor exposure of the femur. Performing the entire procedure through one of these exposures requires either some release of the anterior gluteus medius and minimus or skeletal traction. Skeletal traction has the great disadvantage that a trail reduction is either technically difficult or not performed. Since tissue tension, joint stability, and the absence of prosthetic impingement are critical factors for hip replacement surgery, especially using hard bearings, a trail reduction is essential. As a result, this procedure was designed to be performed without the use of skeletal traction.

Initially, this tissue preserving technique was performed using two exposures. The femoral component preparation and insertion were done through a superior capsulotomy, posterior to the gluteus medius and minimus, and anterior to the short external rotators and posterior capsule. The acetabular component preparation and insertion were done through a Watson Jones interval, inferior to the anterior medius and minimus and deep/lateral to the rectus femoris and psoas. Increasing experience showed that, with angled instruments, both femoral and acetabular component preparation and insertion could be performed through a single incision through a superior capsulotomy.

Description of the Tissue Preserving THA technique

The patient is placed in a lateral position and a 7.5 to 8cm incision is made starting at the tip of the greater trochanter. The skin incision can be longer in heavier patients as necessary. The gluteus maximus fibers are bluntly separated in line with their fibers to reveal the gluteus medius. The posterior border of the gluteus medius is mobilized anterior to reveal the piriformis tendon. The anterior border of the piriformis tendon is developed to reflect the piriformis posteriorly. The insertion of the piriformis is released and repaired as necessary since most uncemented femoral components require removal of the bone that the piriformis tendon inserts upon. The posterior border of the gluteus minimus muscle is developed and the minimus is mobilized anteriorly. A periosteal elevator is used to develop the interval between the minimus tendon and anterior capsule. A blunt homan retractor is placed in between the minimus and anterior capsule and a spiked homan retractor is placed in the ilium to protect the medius and minimus and fully expose the superior hip joint capsule.

A vertical capsulotomy is performed from the trochanteric fossa to the acetabular rim along the course of the piriformis tendon. An anterior capsular flap is developed by tagging the anterior capsule with a suture and incising the capsule along the femoral neck, underneath the minimus tendon and along the anterior-superior acetabular rim. The anterior blunt homan retractor is placed inside the anterior capsule around the anterior femoral neck. Another blunt homan retractor is placed inside the posterior capsule, around the posterior femoral neck. A spike homan retractor is placed in the posterior-superior ilium. These four retractors all of the retraction necessary to perform the procedure (Figure 2).

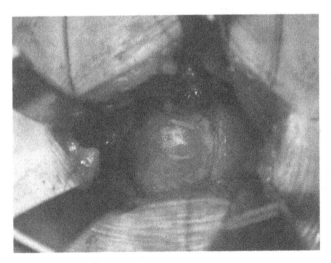

Figure 2:
Figure 2 shows the exposure of a left hip through a superior capsulotomy. The femoral head and labrum are seen in the center of the photograph. The blunt homan in the upper left is inside the anterior capsule, around the femoral neck. The spiked homan in the upper right is in the ilium, underneath the minimus and medius. The spiked homan in the lower right is inside the ilium above the posterior-superior portion of the acetabulum. The blunt homan in the lower left is inside the posterior capsule, around the femoral neck. The entire THA procedure can be performed through this exposure.

The femur is reamed through the superior femoral neck and then the superior portion of the neck is removed with an osteotome to allow the femur to be prepared with broaches. The femoral head and neck are left in situ during this part of the procedure because the head provides stability to the femur during broaching, the neck provides a fulcrum for leverage retractors, and the neck also provides reinforcement to the calcar region to reduce the likelihood of femoral fractures during femoral preparation (Figure 3).

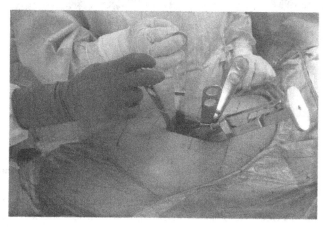

Figure 3:
Figure 3 shows a femoral broach fully inserted through the exposure. The femur is fully prepared through the top of the femoral neck, prior to removal of the femoral head so long as the hip adducts sufficiently to allow this. The femoral head is left in place to stabilize the femur during preparation and to allow leverage retractors (blunt homans) to facilitate exposure.

Once the femur is fully prepared, a skeletal reference frame for surgical navigation is percutaneously affixed to the pelvis and leg length measurement is made. If fluoroscopic navigation is used, fluoroscopic images may be acquired at this point, or before if femoral navigation is employed. The femoral head and neck are then transected, using the blunt homan retractors to protect the surrounding soft tissues. Shanz screws are placed into the head and neck segments and they are excised. If CT based navigation is used, data points on the pelvis and acetabular are now acquired to achieve pelvic registration.

The blunt homan retractors are now placed around the acetabulum anteriorly and posteriorly in the lesser sciatic notch. The entire acetabulum can be seen and remnants of the labrum are excised. A very low profile, 45 degree angled reamer is then used to prepare the acetabulum. A z-shaped acetabular impactor is used to insert the acetabular component with assistance of surgical navigation, with the cup position generally aimed for 41 degrees of abduction and 25 to 30 degrees of anteversion (Figure 4). While acetabular screws are rarely used for fixation, if they are necessary, two methods may be used. The screws may be placed from posterior, just above the edge of the retracted posterior capsule, but this method often requires a slightly longer superficial and fascial incision. The second method allows percutaneous insertion of screws through the Watson-Jones interval, using standard hip arthroscopy cannulas and straight screw insertion instruments.

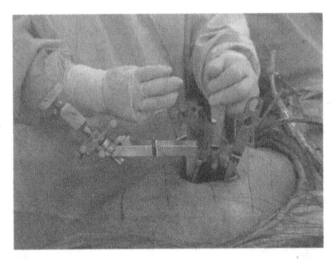

Figure 4:
Figure 4 shows the navigated acetabular impactor during cup insertion. The cup impactor is designed with two 45 degree and one 90 degree angle to allow the cup impactor to exit the incision above the greater trochanter while still allowing impaction of the cup in line with the cup axis.

After the cup is inserted, potentially impinging bone is trimmed, the trial or real alumina acetabular liner is inserted, a trial femoral head is inserted, a trial neck is affixed to the broach, and the trial neck is reduced into the trial head in situ using a bone hook for traction and maximal muscle relaxation. The head and neck are not assembled before reduction because the surrounding soft tissues are so stable that even displacement to allow reduction of a 32mm head may be difficult or cause disruption of surrounding tissues. An intraoperative radiograph may be taken to confirm proper component size and position as necessary. Trial reduction should produce a hip that cannot be dislocated in any direction without traction.

After satisfactory trial reduction, the trial components are removed, the real alumina femoral head is inserted, the real femoral component is inserted, and the femoral neck is again reduced into the femoral head in situ as before. The hip joint capsule is closed and the gluteus minimus and medius return to their native positions when the retractors are removed. The fascia overlying the gluteus maximus is closed prior to subcutaneous and skin closure (Figure 5). Postoperatively, the patient may progress motion and weight bearing without restriction.

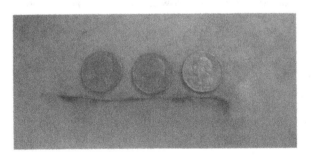

Figure 5:
Figure 5 shows the 8.5cm incision at the completion of the procedure.
The abductors and posterior are fully intact.

Results

Of the 261 total hip arthroplasties, 60 hips have been seen at a minimum of 2 years following surgery, mean 40 months, range 26 to 72 months. The group of 261 hips overall have a mean follow up of 14.5 months. There have been three revisions. One was for failure of osseointegration of a femoral component in a necrotic proximal femur, a second was for malseating of an acetabular liner, treated by proper reinsertion of the liner, and the third was for an acetabular component that displaced at the time of surgery and recognized in the PACU which required prompt revision. Reoperations other than revision were I&D for acute infection in one, I&D without infection in one, ORIF of a post-operative greater trochanteric fracture in one, and ORIF of a greater trochanteric non union in one. There were no dislocations, no bearing fractures, and no radiographic evidence of wear or lysis.

Cup abduction angles in the total hip arthroplasties performed with computer-assisted surgical navigation averaged 41.1 degrees with a range of 35 to 49 degrees and a standard deviation of 2.3 degrees. Cup abduction angles in total hip arthroplasties performed without surgical navigation averaged 42.8 degrees with a range of 26 to 55 degrees and a standard deviation of 4.7 degrees.

Looking specifically at the tissue preserving, minimally invasive hips performed with surgical navigation, complications included one intraoperative trochanteric fracture repaired at the time of surgery, a transverse acetabular fracture during cup impaction recognized during surgery and treated successfully with protected weight bearing. The patient where the acetabular cup displaced at the time of surgery was surgery performed using the minimally invasive technique. That hip was severely dysplastic and in a patient with a body mass index of more than 35. There have been no femur fractures. Analysis of complications as a function of the number of procedures performed, all three surgical complications occurred in the first 43 procedures. The average length of stay for these patients was 3.5 days. By contrast, the patients treated by conventional surgery had a average length of stay of 4.25 days. Most dramatically concerning the use of walking aides, patients who underwent tissue preserving, minimally invasive THA had a mean score of 6.0 (SD 4.3) on a Harris Hip Scale. By contrast, patients who underwent conventional THA had a mean score of 1.86 (SD 2.96).

Discussion

The current study demonstrates that alumina on alumina tha is extremely reliable in a generally young and active patient population. The absence of osteolysis in this series is promising since osteolysis is the most common current cause of failure in total hip arthroplasty. This finding is also encouraging as reports of osteolysis with both electron beam and gamma irradiated polyethylene bearings have been reported already in bearings that have only been available since late 1998. The absence of hip dislocation in this series of 261 consecutive hip replacements is especially reassuring. Concerns that alumina ceramic bearings (with fewer available modular options such as lipped liners and or extra long heads) might lead to greater incidence of instability are clearly unfounded. This may be due, in part, to the femoral neck designs that allow for increased range of motion and the typically larger (32mm or more) bearing diameters used in many of these patients.

Bearing fracture has long been a concern with alumina –on-alumina bearings. While this issue remains a concern, the absence of bearing problems in this series is encouraging. This is especially true given the extreme demands that some of the more active patients subject their hips to. Figure 6 shows the 5 year postoperative radiograph of a patient whose hip as experienced more than 20 million cycles already, that majority of which have been high-impact running activities.

Computer-assisted surgical navigation is performed routinely now and the results of this study show that the use of this technology eliminates malpositioned acetabular cups. There is no other efficient method of achieving this goal. The pelvis moves too much during surgery for any mechanical instrument to be as accurate since the pelvic position during surgery is unknown. Similarly, intraoperative radiographs are often extremely misleading due to deviations from the AP plane.

The use of tissue-preserving, minimally invasive techniques combined with surgical navigation has had a dramatic effect on patient recovery. While length of stay has not dramatically decreased, recovery at 6 weeks is dramatically accelerated. While these techniques can be used for the vast majority of patients, significant deformities or contractures and obesity are factors that may be better addressed with conventional exposures. Of the last 30 patients who underwent primary THA, 24 were performing using minimally invasive techniques. Reasons for conventional techniques were protrusio in 2, severe anteversion from DDH in 2, achondroplasia in one, and morbid obesity in one.

From this preliminary experience, ceramic-ceramic total hip arthroplasty is extremely reliable. Component positioning can be improved with routine use of image-based surgical navigation, and recovery can be greatly facilitated in the majority of primary THA patients by the use of minimally-invasive, tissue preserving techniques.

Acknowledgements: The author wishes to acknowledge Korena Larsen, P.A., Jan Addison, RN, BSN, MEd.

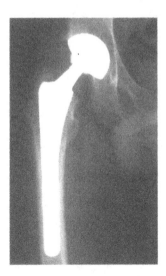

Figure 6:
AP radiograph of a total hip arthroplasty 5 years after implantation. The patient was 46 at the time of surgery and the hip has experienced more than 20 million, mostly high impact cycles as estimated by calculation of stride-length multiplied by distance.

References

1. Barrack R, Castro FP, Jr, Szuszczewicz ES, Schmalzried TP: Analysis of retrieved uncemented porous-coated acetabular components in patients with and without pelvic osteolysis. Orthopaedics, 25(12): 2002.

2. Bizot P, Larrouy M, Witvoet J, Sedel L, Nizard R: Press-fit metal-backed alumina sockets: A minimum 5-year follow-up study. Clin Orthop, 379:134-142, 2000.

3. Boutin P: The classic: Total hip arthroplasty using a ceramic prosthesis. Clin Orthop, 379: 3-11, 2000.

4. Dorlot JM. J. Biomed Mater Res 1989 Dec 23(A3 Suppl):299-310.

5. Digas G, Kärrholm J, Thanner J, Malchau H, Herberts P: Highly Cross-Linked Polyethylene in Hip Arthroplasty. Randomized Study Using Radiostereometry (Preliminary Report). 31st Open Scientific Meeting & 9th Combined Open Meeting of the Hip Society & AAHKS, New Orleans, Louisiana, February 8, 2003.

6. DiGioia AM, Plakseychuk AY, Levisoin TJ, Jaramaz B. Mini-incision technique for total hip arthroplasty with navigation. J. Arthroplasty. 2003 Feb/18(2):123-128.

7. Eickmann TH, Clarke IC, Gustafson GA. Squeaking in a Ceramic on Ceramic Total Hip. In Bioceramics in Joint Arthroplasty. Zippel H and Dietrich M editors. Steinkopff Darmstadt Publishers. p187-192, 2003.

8. Endo MM, Barbour PS, Barton DC, Fisher J, Tipper JL, Ingham E, Stone MH: Comparative wear and wear debris under three different counterface conditions of crosslinked and non-crosslinked ultra high molecular weight polyethylene. Biomed Mater Eng, 11(1): 23-35, 2001.

9. Fischer J, Besong AA, Firkins PJ, Barbour PSM, Nevelos JE, Tripper JL, Stone MH, Ingham E: Comparative wear and debris generation in UHMWPE on ceramic, metal on metal and ceramic on ceramic hip prostheses. 46th Annual Meeting of the Orthopaedic Research Society, Orlando, FL, March 12-15, 2002.

10. Garino JP: Modern ceramic-on-ceramic total hip systems in the United States: Early results. Clin Orthop, 379:41-47, 2000.

11. Hamadouche M, Boutin P, Daussange J, Bolander M, and Sedel L. Alumina-on-Alumina Total Hip Arthroplasty: A Minimum 18.5-Year Follow-up Study. Journal of Bone and Joint Surgery 84A(1): 69-77, 2002.

12. Heck DA, Partridge CM, Reuben JD, Lanzer WL, Lewis CG, Keating EM: Prosthetic component failures in hip arthroplasty surgery. J Arthroplasty, 10(5):575-580, 1995.

13. Mallory TH, Lombardi AV, Jr, Fada RA, Herrington SM, Eberle RW: Dislocation after total hip arthroplasty using the anterolateral abductor split approach. Clin Orthop, 358:166-172, 1999.

14. Martell J. Cross-Linkage: Another Strategy. 6th Annual Alternative Bearings Symposium, San Fransisco, September 22, 2003.

15. Murphy SB: Ceramic-ceramic bearings in THA: The new gold standard – in the affirmative. Orthopaedics, 25(9):933-934, 2002.

16. Murphy SB, Bierbaum B. Eberle RW. American Experience with Alumina Ceramic-Ceramic Bearings in Total Hip Arthroplasty. In Bioceramics in Joint Arthroplasty. Zippel H and Dietrich M editors. Steinkopff Darmstadt Publishers. p157-162, 2003.

17. Murphy SB and Deshmukh R. Clinical Results of Computer-Assisted Total Hip Arthroplasty. International Society of Computer Assisted Orthopedic Surgery. 2003.

18. Reis M. Cross-Linked Polyethylene: To be or not to be. 6th Annual Alternative Bearings Symposium, San Fransisco, September 22, 2003.

19. Timmerman I, Murphy S. Fatigue Resistance of Ceramic Liners to the Physiological Loading Under Conditions of Impingement. International Society of Technology in Arthroplasty, San Fransisco, September 24, 2003.

Alternative Wear Couples Solutions/
Pro's and Con's

3.1 Phase Transformation in Zirconia Heads after THA Myth or Reality?

J. Caton, J.-P. Bouraly, P. Reynaud and Z. Merabet

Introduction

From 1985 to 2001, about 400 000 zircon heads Prozyr™ had been implanted for total hip arthroplasties (THA). In FRANCE following an abnormal rate of ball fractures, concerning the introduction of the tunnel Furnace (TH), instead of the batch furnace method (BH) the manufacture of zircon heads was stopped in August 2001. Following the works of ALLAIN et al., another controversy arose regarding zircon heads, presenting an abnormal rate of polywear with osteolysis secondary according to the authors: "an increased roughness of the head by phase transformation with tearing off of grains". This hypothesis was corroborated by HARAGUCHI et al. (2001) reporting on 2 explanted heads. We were prompted to verify this hypothesis.

Patient and Method

In 2002 we explanted three 22.2 mm zircon heads Prozyr™ on account of recurrent dislocation which we compared with one new zircon head Prozyr™ and with one alumina head (diam. 28) also explanted for loosening and one new alumina head using the same protocol as HARAGUCHI et al.

Result

The percentage of monoclinic phase found was always very low and below 10% (3 to 10%) on the explanted heads. The roughness values (Ra) remained also very low with an Ra of 0,01μm whatever the head, zircon or ceramic, new or explanted, without grains pull out and without any notable structural modification, the average grain size of the femoral heads remaining in accordance with the ISO norm 13 356 (1977).

Discussion

IC CLARKE (2003) selected, among 23 explanted zircon heads, 3 heads at 2.8 and 10 years follow-up. The heads at 2 and 10 years did not show any phase transformation nor any surface lesions. On the explanted head at 8 years, a large monoclinic phase transformation was observed. In our study, on the 3 heads explanted we did not observe any significant monoclinic phase transformation, since it remained below 10% without grain pull out nor increased roughness. It is possible that the behaviour of the 22.2 mm Prozyr™ zircon heads is different from 28mm zircon heads, whether fractures are concerned (since no fracture with 22.2 mm head was observed following TH oven baking) or the monoclinic phase transformation.

Conclusion

The outcome is important for all patients with a zircon head THA. It is quite obvious that surveillance should be continued. In the immediate and at middle term, we can conclude that the monoclinic phase transformation rate is low for explanted Prozyr™ zircon heads and allows one to suppose that the manufacturing quality of heads is good, particularly as regards 22.225 mm diameters.

3.2 Charnley-Kerboull Total Hip Arthroplasty Combining Zirconia on Polyethylene A Minimum 2-Year Follow-Up Prospective Study

M. Hamadouche, F. Madi, L. Kerboull, J.-P. Courpied and M. Kerboull

Introduction

Polyethylene wear and polyethylene particles induced periprosthetic osteolysis remains currently the major limitation to the long-term performance of total hip arthroplasty. To reduce polyethylene wear, P. Boutin introduced alumina ceramic femoral heads in the early 1970's. However, the relative brittle nature of alumina was responsible for a high rate of fracture. Improvement in the manufacturing process with a low grain size and grain distribution dramatically decreased the risk of crack propagation and rate of fracture. Despite these improvements, the use of 22.2-mm diameter alumina ceramic femoral head is not recommended in Europe.

Zirconia ceramic femoral heads were introduced in orthopaedics in 1985 because of the high strength and fracture toughness of the material that would reduce the risk for fracture. Moreover, the physical properties of the material were recently improved with the introduction of hot isostatic pressure (HIP) process. These mechanical properties have allowed the use of 22.2 mm diameter femoral heads. Also, zirconia has a high scratch resistance. A number of in-vitro studies have reported a reduced rate of polyethylene wear articulating against zirconia. Few clinical studies with controversial results have been published. At the authors' institution, Charnley-Kerboull prostheses have been used since 1972. The survival of the prosthesis at 20 years with revision as the end-point was over 80%, wear of the polyethylene cup and osteolysis being the main cause for revision.

To investigate the alleged decreased wear of polyethylene articulating with zirconia, an open prospective clinical trial was started in 1997 to evaluate the clinical and radiologic performances of this combination in total hip arthroplasty. The aim of this study was to report on a short series of Charnley-Kerboull total hip arthroplasties combining zirconia femoral heads with polyethylene with a minimum 2-year follow-up.

Materials and Methods

Between January 1997 and June 1999, 51 patients had 55 total hip replacements, performed by the senior author (M.K.). There were 30 females (33 hips) and 21 males (22 hips) in this series. The average age of the patients at the time of the index arthroplasty was 52.5 ± 12 years (range, 25 to 76 years). The mean weight of the patients was 66 ± 10 Kg (range, 43 to 91 Kg) and height 167 ± 8.6 cm (range, 142 to 189 cm). The mean body mass index of the series was 23.9 ± 3.4 (range, 18 to 33.5). The right hip was operated on in 31 patients and the left in 18, whereas 3 patients had bilateral replacement. Initial diagnoses are summarized in Table 1. Eleven of the 55 hips had had a total hip replacement before the index arthroplasty.

Total replacement was performed through a lateral approach with a trochanteric osteotomy in all cases. The technique has been previously reported in details.

Table1:
Initial diagnosis.

Underlying disease	Number of hips	Percent
Primary osteoarthritis	27	49.1
Congenital hip dysplasia	16	29.1
Post-traumatic osteoarthritis	4	7.3
Avascular necrosis	3	5.5
Rheumatoid arthritis	2	3.6
Ankylosing spondylitis	2	3.6
Vilonodular synovitis	1	1.8
TOTAL	55	100

A zirconia on polyethylene combination was used in all patients, and implants were of Charnley-Kerboull design (Fig. 1). The femoral stem was made of polished stainless steel orthinox (Legend®, Benoist-Girard, Howmedica, Herouville Saint-Clair, France). The socket was made of cross-linked polyethylene (Duration®, Benoist-Girard, Howmedica, Herouville Saint-Clair, France). Cross-linking was developed by sterilizing GUR 415 ultra-high molecular weight polyethylene with 3.0 Mrad of gamma irradiation in an atmosphere of nitrogen and then subjecting the packaged components to an annealing cycle to promote further cross-linking via a radical quenching mechanism. Both components were fixed according to a second-generation technique using CMW type 1 bone cement (Depuy 1 Bone cement, Exeter, Devon, England). This cement contained baryum sulfate as a radio-opacifying agent, and was zirconium oxide free.

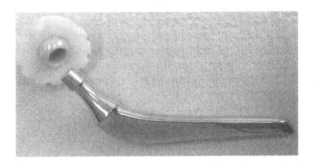

Figure 1:
Charnley-Kerboull total hip arthroplasty combining zirconia on polyethylene.

The 22.2 mm femoral head was made of yttria-stabilized tetragonal zirconia polycrystal ceramic (Y-TZP) processed according to the hot isostatic pressure procedure (Prozyr®, Norton Demarquest, Evreux, France). The main characteristics of the material as indicated by the manufacturer comparatively to International Standards Organization (ISO 13356) are summarized in Table 2. The zirconia femoral head was secured to the femoral stem through a Morse taper that had an angle of 11°25 in 27 hips and 5°40 in the remaining 28 hips.

Table2:
Physical and chemical properties of zirconia ceramics

Property	ISO 13356	Prozyr® (Norton Demarquest)
ZrO_2 (%)	> 94.2	>
Y_2O_3 (%)	5.1 ± 0.3	5.1 ± 0.3
Density (g/cm³)	> 6.00	> 6.08
Mean grain size (μm)	< 0.5	< 0.5
Surface finish (Ra, μm)	-	> 600
Compressive strength (MPa)	2000	-
Young's modulus (GPa)	210	-
Bending strength (Mpa)	> 900	> 1500
Biaxial strength	-	> 600
Fracture toughness Mpa m$^{1/2}$	-	8-10
Monoclinic phase		

Postoperative treatment included anticoagulation therapy, systemic antibiotics and non-steroidal anti-inflammatory drugs (ketoprofen, 100 milligrams per day) to prevent heterotopic ossification. Immediate postoperative passive motion exercises of the operated joint were undertaken. Passive motion exercises were therapist assisted and were pursued until active motion of the hip was possible. Patients were free to walk with two supports after three days. Full weight bearing was usually allowed after six weeks.

Cystic or scalloped lesions greater than two millimeters in diameter around the prosthetic components that were not present on the immediate postoperative radiograph were defined as osteolysis. Statistical analysis was performed using non-parametric tests. Significance was defined as a p value of less than 0.05 (StatView 5.0 Statistical Software, SAS Institute Inc., USA).

Results

All 51 patients (55 hips) had a minimal two-year follow-up. No patient was lost to follow-up and no patient died during the study period. The mean follow-up of the series was 32 ± 6 months (range, 24 to 48 months).

No patient had infection, and no prosthesis dislocation occurred. No other complication was recorded in this series, including the absence of femoral head fracture. No patient was revised.

The mean Merle d'Aubigné functional hip score increased from 12.1 ± 2.7 preoperatively to 17.9 ± 0.1 at last follow-up (Wilcoxon rank test, $p < 0.001$). Functional hip score parameters at last follow-up compared with preoperative data are presented in (Figure 2.) Fifty-one hips (47 patients) were rated as excellent, 3 hips (3 patients) as very good, and one hip (one patient) as good. Fifty patients (54 hips) had no pain in the operated joint, whereas one patient (one hip) had a moderate pain not restricting their activity level. Forty-eight patients (52 hips) had a normal gait, whereas three patients (3 hips) needed one cane for long distance walking. These three patients belonged to the revision group. The mean range of flexion of the series was 115 ± 15 degrees (range, 90 to 130 degrees).

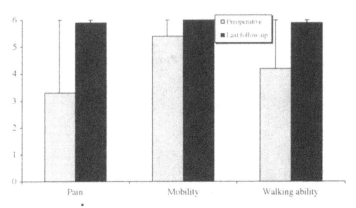

Figure 2:
Preoperative and last follow-up Merle d'Aubigné hip score parameters.

The mean abduction angle of the socket was 41.9 ± 5.7 degrees (range, 29 to 52 degrees). The mean distance of the most medial point of the prosthetic cup to the vertical teardrop line was 3.7 ± 1.9 mm (range, 0.8 to 8.3 mm), whereas the lower point of the prosthetic cup liner to the horizontal teardrop line was 2.7 ± 3.3 mm (range, -4 to 12 mm). At the latest follow-up, there was no significant difference in any of these parameters (p > 0.5).

Radiolucent lines less than 1 mm thick were observed in 2 hips on the acetabular side in Zone II, and in 2 hips in Zone II and III. On the femoral side, radiolucent lines in Zone VI and VII were observed in 4 hips. No case of stem migration was recorded in this series. Therefore, according to the criteria used in this study, no implant loosening occurred.

Wear, as measured radiographicaly on plain anteroposterior view of the pelvis, was always less than 0.5 millimeter (accuracy of the caliper) at the latest follow-up.

Lytic lesions in Zone VII of the femur were recorded in 19 of the 55 hips (34.5%). These lesions appeared as either calcar resorption or endosteal cysts in the proximal and medial region of the femur. They measured less than 1 cm², and always occurred between the first and second year. They were non-progressive between the second year and last follow-up (Fig. 3 and 4).

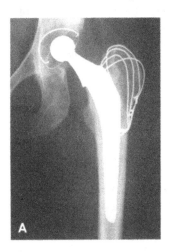

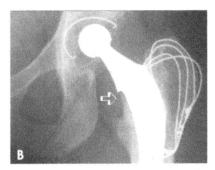

Figure 3:
3a: Postoperative radiograph of a 58 years old male that underwent total hip arthroplasty for primary osteoarthritis.
3b: Radiograph made at 29-month follow-up showing calcar resorption (arrow).

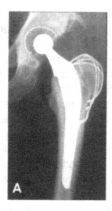
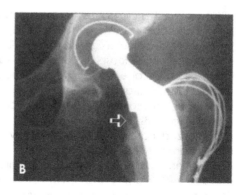

Figure 4:
4a: Postoperative radiograph of a 31 years old male that underwent total hip arthroplasty for post-traumatic avscular necrosis of the femoral head.
4b: Radiograph made at 27-month follow-up showing endosteal lytic lesion in Zone VII of the femur.

Preoperative parameters were tested to evaluate their predictive value on the occurrence of lytic lesions in Zone VII of the femur. Gender did not significantly influence the rate of osteolyis (9 cases of 33 hips in females versus 10 cases of 22 hips in males, Fisher exact probability, p = 0.25). Neither did the age at the time of arthroplasty or body mass index (respectively, Fisher exact probability, p = 0.37 and p = 0.29). The occurrence of lytic lesions was not significantly different according to the angle of the Morse taper (16 cases of the 27 hips with a Morse taper of 11°25 versus 8 cases of the 28 hips with a Morse taper of 5°40, Fisher exact probability, p = 0.40). Lytic lesions in Zone VII of the femur were recorded in 2 of the 11 hips that belonged the revision total hip arthroplasty group versus 17 of the 45 primary hip replacements. The difference was not significant (Fisher exact probability, p = 0.30).

Discussion

Surgical grade zirconia ceramic was introduced in orthopaedics in 1985. The metastable nature of zirconia required the use of yttria to enable stability of the material in its tetragonal allotropic phase. The biocompatibilty and the low magnitude of inflammatory response induced by zirconia particles have been demonstrated by several studies.

Most of the reported in vitro studies demonstrated a lower rate of polyethylene wear articulating with zirconia when compared to metal, with either bovine serum or water as a lubricant. The wear rates were comparable to those obtained with alumina on polyethylene. These results were confirmed in an in vivo study performed in a canine model by Hamada et al. comparing alumina versus zirconia articulating with polyethylene.

Clinical results published in the literature are sparse and controversial. To the best of the authors' knowledge only two clinical studies have reported favorable results with the use of either 28 or 22 mm zirconia femoral heads at short-term follow-up. The wear rate in these studies was less than 0.1 mm/year.

However, other clinical results have not been so favorable. Allain et al. reported on a consecutive series of 100 total hip arthroplasties using 28 mm zirconia femoral heads articulating with polyethylene. At a mean follow-up of 5.8 years, 13% of acetabular loosening and 47.5% radiolucent lines at the cement bone interface on the acetabular side occurred, whereas on the femoral side 2.5% of femoral loosening and 21.7% of radiolucent lines at the cement bone interface were observed. Moreover, a 20% rate of calcar lysis was seen. The survival rate at 8 years was 63%. Histological analysis revealed zirconia particles. The authors hypothesized that zirconia particles of low purity occurred from cement opacifier rather than from the articulating surface. Recently Kim et al. reported on a series of 70 patients that had one stage bilateral total hip arthroplasty using zirconia on one side and chrome cobalt on the other combining with a polyethylene socket. The mean follow-up of the series was 6.4 years. The authors did not find a significant difference in wear of the polyethylene socket, although a tendency towards higher rates was observed with zirconia heads within the 3 first postoperative years. Finally, Haraguchi et al. reported on two cases of phase transformation of retrieved zirconia femoral heads. One head was retrieved at revision due to recurrent dislocation after six years and the other because of failure of the locking mechanism of the polyethylene liner after three years. The monoclinic content of the zirconia ceramics rose from 1% to about 30% on the surface of the heads. Surface electron microscopy revealed numerous craters indicating extraction of the zirconia ceramics at the surface. Surface roughness increased from an initial value of 0.006 mm up to 0.12 μm.

The absence of correlation between hip simulator studies and clinical results could be interpreted in the light of Lu et al. findings. These authors have shown that major frictional heating was observed in vitro when testing zirconia against polyethylene. This phenomenon was responsible for proteins lubricant precipitation. The resultant protein layer between the femoral head and polyethylene socket could protect the bearing surfaces from wear. The maximum temperatures reached in vivo are likely much lower than those observed in the hip simulator as patients do not walk so fast so long. In this respect, polyethylene wear is probably underestimated by hip simulator.

In the current clinical study, although zirconia was used in optimal conditions, including a single experienced surgeon, hot isostatic pressure process, a zirconium free cement, and 22-mm head, we observed moderate osteolysis of the proximal femur in one third of the hips at 2 to 4-year follow-up. This phenomenon could be interpreted as running-in wear or as the first steps of major wear that will increase with longer term follow-up. The authors have decided to quit the implantation of zirconia femoral heads until long-term follow-up results have been obtained.

This study emphases that the projection of the in vitro results of a material should be projected with extreme caution to the in vivo behavior.

References

1. Allain J, Le Mouel S, Goutallier D, Voisin MC (1999) Poor eight-year survival of cemented zirconia-polyethylene total hip replacements. J Bone Joint Surg Br 81-B:835-842.
2. Boutin P (1972) Arthroplastie totale de la hanche par prothèse en alumine fittée. Etude expérimentale et premières applications cliniques. Rev Chir Orthop 58:229-246.
3. Cales B (2000) Zirconia as a sliding material: histologic, laboratory, and clinical data. Clin Orthop 379:94-112.
4. Caton J, Merabet Z, Reynaud P, Termanian PJ (2001) Etude comparative de l'usure de deux séries de prothèses totales de hanche (tête 22,225 mm, zircone/PE et métal/PE). Proceedings of the 76th SoFCOT, Paris, France.
5. Christel P (1992): Biocompatibility of surgical-grade dense polycrystalline alumina. Clin Orthop 282:10-18.
6. Clarke IC, Gustafson A (2000) Clinical and hip simulator comparisons of ceramic-on-polyethylene and metal-on-polyethylene wear. Clin Orthop 379:34-40.
7. De Lee J, Charnley J (1976) Radiological demarcation of cemented sockets in total hip replacement. Clin Orthop 121: 20-32.
8. Derbyshire B, Fisher J, Dowson D, Hardaker C, Brummitt K (1994) Comparative study of the wear of UHMWPE with zirconia ceramic and stainless steel femoral heads in artificial hip joints. Med Eng Phys 16:229-236.
9. Goldsmith AA, Dowson D (1999) A multi-station hip joint simulator study of theperformance of 22 mm diameter zirconia-ultra-high molecular weight polyethylene total replacement hip joints. Proc Inst Mech Eng 213: 77-90.
10. Goldsmith AA, Dowson D, Isaac GH, Lancaster JG (2000) A comparative joint simulator study of the wear of metal-on-metal and alternative material combinations in hip replacements. Proc Inst Mech Eng 214:39-47.
11. Goodman S, Huie P, Song Y, et al. (1997) Loosening and osteolysis of cemented joint arthroplasties. A biologic spectrum. Clin Orthop 337:149-163.
12. Gruen TA, McNeice GM, Amstutz HC (1979) "Modes of failure" of cemented stem-type femoral components: a radiographic analysis of loosening. Clin Orthop 141: 17-27.
13. Hamada Y, Horiuchi T, Sano Y, Usui I (1999) The wear of a polyethylene socket articulating with a zirconia ceramic femoral head in canine total hip arthroplasty. J Biomed Mater Res 48: 301-308.
14. Haraguchi K, Sugano N, Nishii T, Miki, H, Oka, K, Yoshikawa, H (2001) Phase transformation of a zirconia ceramic head after total hip arthroplasty. J Bone Joint Surg Br 83:996-1000.
15. Jiranek WA, Machado M, Jasty M, et al. (1993) Production of cytokines around loosened cemented acetabular components. Analysis with immunohistochemical techniques and in situ hybridization. J Bone Joint Surg Am 75: 863-879.
16. Kim YH, Kim JS, Cho SH (2001) A comparison of polyethylene wear in hips with cobalt-chrome or zirconia heads. A prospective, randomised study. J Bone Joint Surg Br 83:742-750.
17. Kumar P, Oka M, Ikeuchi K, et al. (1991) Low wear rate of UHMWPE against zirconia ceramic (Y-PSZ) in comparison to alumina ceramic and SUS 316L alloy. J Biomed Mater Res 25:813-828.
18. Lancaster JG, Dowson D, Isaac GH, Fisher J (1997) The wear of ultra-high molecular weight polyethylene sliding on metallic and ceramic counterfaces representative of current femoral surfaces in joint replacement. Proc Inst Mech Eng 211:17-24.
19. Livermore J, Ilstrup D, Morrey B (1990) Effect of femoral head size on wear of the polyethylene acetabular component. J Bone Joint Surg Am 72:518-528.
20. Lu Z, McKellop H (1997) Frictional heating of bearing materials tested in a hip joint wear simulator. Proc Inst Mech Eng 211: 101-108.

21. Lu Z, McKellop H, Liao P, Benya P (1999) Potential thermal artifacts in hip joint wear simulators. J Biomed Mater Res 48:458-464.
22. Maloney WJ, Jasty M, Harris WH, Galante, JO, Callaghan, JJ (1990) Endosteal erosion in association with stable uncemented femoral components. J Bone Joint Surg Am 72:1025-1034.
23. Merle d'Aubigné R (1970) Cotation chiffreé de la fonction de la hanche. Rev Chir Orthop 56: 481-486.
24. Piconi C, Burger W, Richter HG, et al. (1998) Y-TZP ceramics for artificial joint replacements. Biomaterials 19:1489-1494.
25. Semlitsch M, Willert HG (1997) Clinical wear behaviour of ultra-high molecular weight polyethylene cups paired with metal and ceramic ball heads in comparison to metal-on-metal pairings of hip joint replacements. Proc Inst Mech Eng 211:73-88.

3.3 Highly Cross-linked Polyethylene – A New Option in Tribology of THA

L. Rabenseifner

Introduction

Highly cross-linked polyethylene Durasul was introduced at our hospital in March 1999. In vitro results regarding wear behaviour from different laboratories are very encouraging. Durasul polyethylene inlays showed after 27 million cycles no measurable wear in an AMTI hip simulator study. The ultra-low wear was masked by the minute fluid uptake from the serum. To date, only few in vivo results exist and show a tendency that Durasul resists to wear better than conventional polyethylene [1]. Thus, there is still a demand for investigations using early wear detection methods in order to expose a minimum number of patients to the risk of material failure.

We conducted two Durasul clinical investigations:
1. a prospective clinical study aiming measurements of femoral head penetration into polyethylene liners using PolyWare edge detection algorithm [2].
2. a retrieval study aiming the following analysis in each explanted liner made of Durasul Polyethylene:
   a) Surface analysis with light and electron scan microscope.
   b) Histological investigation of periprosthetic tissue.

Materials and method

1. Prospective investigation of penetration

Investigation about the performance of Durasul was designed as an ongoing prospective study. The study comprises 295 patients. A group of 10 patients with total hip arthroplasty using conventional polyethylene was used as control.

The implants used in this study are cemented anatomical stems (Optan) in combination with a 28 mm CoCr metal head, a press-fit titanium cup (Fitmore) with a highly cross-linked polyethylene liner (Durasul). In the control group, the same implants were used, except for the liner where a conventional UHMWPE was used. The follow-ups were done at 3 months post-operative, 1 year, 2 years, and each year after.

To measure and track penetration of the femoral head into the polyethylene liner, we used the PolyWare algorithm. This 3D technique uses digitized x–rays of a standard A/P view (Fig. 1a) and a shoot–through lateral view (Fig. 1b), which is taken in an angled position of 90 degrees in comparison to the standard A/P view. All x–rays were scanned at 100% magnification with a resolution of 250 dpi. The software reconstructs in 3D the center of the ball head and the cup, and calculates the relative displacement of the two centers in all directions. The accuracy of this method is ± 0.15 mm.

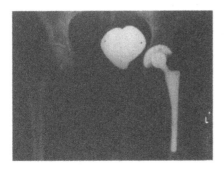
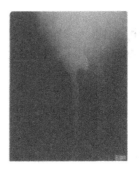

Figure 1a:
Standard a/p –view with the beam centered on the symphysis.

Figure 1b:
Shoot-through lateral.

2. Retrieval study

To date, we reviewed and documented 8 retrieved Durasul liners that were explanted after periods ranging from 3 to 43 months (Table 1):
Two cases due to a trauma after 3 and 5 months, three due to infection after 5, 14 and 26 months, one due to loosening of the cup as a result of an intra-operative technical problem after 10 months, one revision because of periarticular ossifications after 15 months and one following recurrent luxation after 43 months.

In all cases, the periprosthetic tissue was histologically analyzed in collaboration with Prof. H.G. Willert.

Table 1:
Overview of analyzed explants.

	Reason for Revision	**Time in vivo**
Case 1	Fracture posttraumatic	3 months
Case 2	Fracture posttraumatic	5 months
Case 3	Infection	5 months
Case 4	Fracture, loosening	10 months
Case 5	Infection	14 months
Case 6	Ossification	15 months
Case 7	Infection	26 months
Case 8	Luxation posttraumatic	43 months

All explants' articulating surfaces were investigated using light microscopy, and some of them were also investigated by scanning electron microscopy.

Due to the anticipated ultra low amount of wear and hence ultra low material loss, accumulation of surface changes (i.e. scratches) was expected on the articulating surfaces.

By means of remelting experiments (e.g. exposition of polyethylene to heat above the crystalline melting point which initiates the memory effect of UHMWPE [3, 4]), it is possible to distinguish surface changes due to wear from surface changes due to other mechanisms. Hence, surface investigations with light microscopy were performed before and after melting.

Results

Measurements of penetration using PolyWare

The penetration of the ball head into the polyethylene liner was measured as described above.

Due to the well-described bedding-in and creep phenomena, which take place first few years after implantation, the results in terms of penetration do not differ significantly between highly cross-linked polyethylene Durasul and the conventional polyethylene. A trend, however, shows that Durasul penetration values are getting smaller than penetrations in conventional polyethylene. The steady state is being settled, after which penetration will be interpreted as wear.

Retrieval study

In general, all histological examinations of periprosthetic tissue revealed extremely low deposition of Durasul polyethylene particles (Figure 2). In comparison with histological findings in conventional polyethylene, the amount of Durasul polyethylene wear particles observed was extremely little. In all cases, there were no signs of any biological reaction.

Case 4 was a special one: this patient has undergone his second revision surgery and before implanting a Durasul liner (2nd revision), the patient had a conventional polyethylene liner in place. In this case, more polyethylene particles were observed. Case 2 showed also extremely low deposition of Durasul polyethylene particles. However, the particles were very large (about 50 mm). This is due to a typical impingement after a proximal femoral fracture.

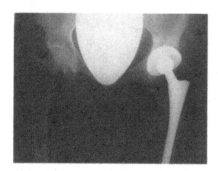 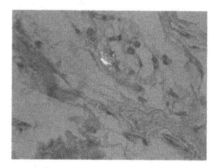

Figure 2a:
Post-op A/P x-ray of Case 3.

Figure 2b:
HE pol 100x Case 3
Extremely low deposition of polyethylene particles.

As wear is supposed to be extremely low with Durasul, more and stronger initial surface changes than with conventional polyethylene are visible (Figure 3).

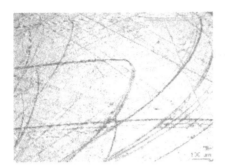

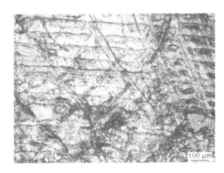

Figure 3a:
Polished (worn) conventional Liner after
6 months in vivo.

Figure 3b:
Scratched Durasul Liner after 15 months
in vivo.

Due to the memory effect of highly cross-linked UHMWPE, exposition to heat above the crystalline melting point enables the reconfiguration of the molecular chains. Flattened machining marks reappear after melting. Scars and scratches disappear, as long as they constitute plastic deformation only without any loss of material (Figure 4).

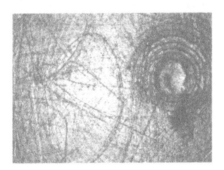

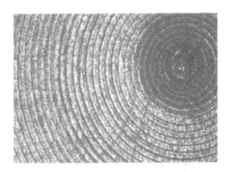

Figure 4a:
Durasul surface as retrieved after 10 months
in vivo.

Figure 4b:
Durasul surface after melting.

Worn machining marks and scratches due to wear (i.e. loss of material) do not reappear after melting. In cases 7 and 8 where the retrievals were obtained after an implantation time of more than 2 years (26 and 43 months respectively), the articulating surfaces showed some signs of minute wear in the loaded area.

Discussion

In the 70's, H.G. Willert described the so-called particle disease, which lead to periprothetic osteolysis in total hip replacement [5].

Liberation of wear particles causes biological reactions, a so-called aggressive, inflammatory fibrous tissue response. Late aseptic implant loosening remains today the major problem in the lifespan of joint replacement. The consequence of evidence-based medicine must be to reduce wear. After 27 million cycles in vitro, Durasul, a highly cross-linked polyethylene, shows a drastic wear reduction. Wear was not measurable due to fluid uptake. This encouraging finding is predictable for an important reduction of in vivo wear and hence a substantial drop of osteolysis risks.

As the short-term (few first years post-op) penetration rate is the combination of bedding-in, creep and wear, the penetration results do not differ significantly between Durasul and conventional polyethylene. A trend is, however, observed and suggests that penetration in case of Durasul started leveling-off and reaching a steady state. This observed trend is in line with published information by the Gothenburg group in 2003 [1]. The 2-year wear as measured by RSA showed a significant lower value in Durasul as compared to conventional polyethylene in the standing position. In the supine position, a trend that Durasul wears less than conventional polyethylene was also observed. According to P. Devane, the penetration rate for conventional polyethylene levels-off to a steady state using his algorithm (PolyWare) around 5 years post-op.

The histological examinations confirm the excellent results known from AMTI hip simulator tests of the MGH in Boston. In all cases, we found an extremely low deposition of polyethylene particles and no biological reaction like macrophages or foreign body giant cells.

The remelting experiments are showing mainly plastic deformation without loss of polyethylene material. After two years or more in vivo and in the 2 cases where machining marks did not reappear following remelting, the first visible signs of wear in the loaded area suggest a yearly wear rate of about 5 mm, since the height of the machining marks is 3-7 μm. The findings confirm the very low amount of wear until 43 months in vivo. For comparison, a good conventional polyethylene should have 0.2 mm wear after two years in vivo.

These results encourage us to continue implanting highly cross-linked polyethylene. The retrieval investigations and radiological analysis will be continued.

References

1. Digas G et al, RSA evaluation of wear of conventional versus highly cross-linked polyethylene acetabular components in vivo. 49th Annual Meetings ORS, p. 1430, 2003.
2. Devane, P. A., Bourne, R. B. et al.: Measurement of polyethylene wear in acetabular components inserted with and without cement. CORR, 319: 303 – 316, 1995.
3. Muratoglu OK et al, Surface analysis of early retrieved acetabular polyethylene liners: A comparison of standard and highly crosslinked polyethylenes, 48th Annual Meeting ORS, p. 1029, 2002.
4. Rieker C et al, In vivo tribological performance of 21 highly crosslinked ultra high molecular weight polyethylene inserts, Rivista di Patologia della Apparato Locomotore Vol. II- Fasc.1 /2, p 47-51, 2003.
5. Willert HG, Semlitsch M, Reactions of the articular capsule to wear products of artificial joint prostheses. J Biomed Mater Res 11(2), 157-164, 1977.

3.4 The Crosslinked Ultra-high Molecular Weight Polyethylene: Risk and Limitation

L. Costa, P. Bracco and E. M. Brach del Prever

Introduction

In the past three decades the majority of the implanted orthopedic prostheses included a bearing component made of ultrahigh molecular weight polyethylene (UHMWPE) articulating against a femoral metallic or ceramic ball or a metallic tibial plateau. Wear of the polyethylene bearing surfaces produces abrasion particles [1], often causing a foreign body response that may lead to bone resorption (osteolysis) and loosening of the components, and thereby limiting the life expectancy of hip prostheses. Thus, improving the wear resistance of the polyethylene can substantially extend the clinical life span of total hip prostheses.

The majority of polyethylene components has been sterilized by gamma irradiation in the presence of air, with doses between 25 and 40 kGy. However, oxygen that was present in the polyethylene when it was irradiated, or that diffused into the polyethylene during shelf storage and/or in vivo, could react with the free radicals that were generated by the radiation, causing oxidative degradation that lowered the molecular mass, increased the density, stiffness and brittleness, and reduced the fracture strength and elongation to failure [2-3]. Any of these changes could adversely affect the wear resistance of the polyethylene [4-5]. In contrast, in absence of oxygen, the free radicals generated during radiation sterilization could form crosslinked polyethylene molecules [6-7], and crosslinking has been shown to markedly improve the wear resistance of polyethylene acetabular cups in laboratory wear simulators [8-11] and in clinical studies [12-16]. Consequently, orthopaedic researches were directed to the development of an UHMWPE implant that has the resistance to oxidation of the unirradiated polyethylene while possesses optimum level of crosslinking to improve its wear resistance.

Risk

Irradiation of UHMWPE with high energy radiation (gamma or electron beam) leads to physico-chemical modifications of the polymer, which can be summarized as follows:

a) Chemical changes. The energy of e-beam or gamma radiation is some order of magnitude higher than that of C-C and C-H bonds. Thus, irradiation causes bond scissions (scheme 1, reaction 1 and 2) and formation of alkyl macro-radicals which can survive for years after irradiation. Some of the radicals decay giving cross-liking (scheme 1, reaction 4), trans-vinylene double bonds (scheme 1, reaction 3) and elimination of vinyl double bonds with further cross-linking (scheme 1, reaction 5).

b) Physical changes. Irradiation leads to a minimum increase in cristallinity, due to bond scissions, with a slight variation of the maximum of the melting peak, originated from a change in the lamellae thicknesses.

c) Mechanical properties. Physical and chemical modifications of the polymeric structure induce also changes in the mechanical behaviour. Cross-linking leads to an increase in the Young modulus, while the formation of trans-vinylene double bonds give reason of a decrease in the elongation and tensile stress at failure.

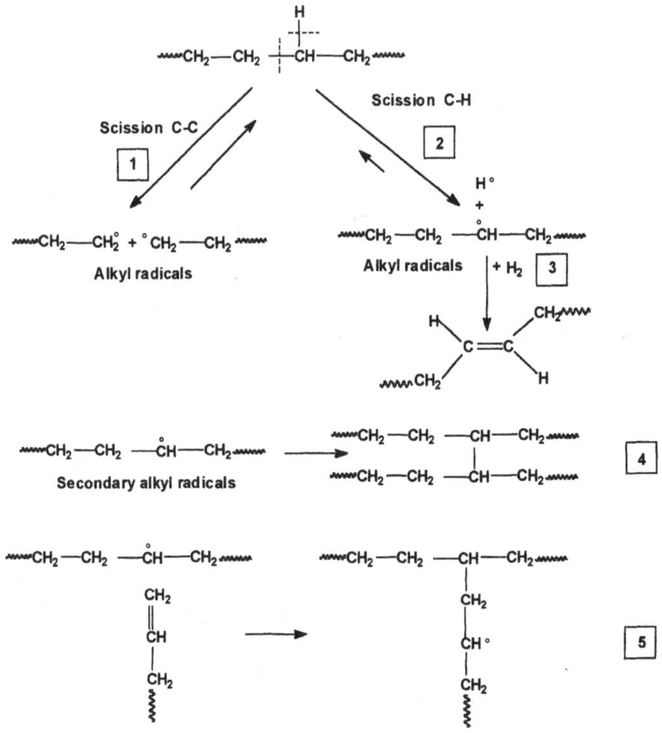

Scheme 1:
The crosslinked process by high energy radiation.

Each producer adopt one of the following techniques: application of the maximum radiation dose compatible with the mechanical properties specified by international standards (ASTM and ISO), in order to highly cross-link the polymer and maximize the abrasion resistance or use of a lower radiation dose, enhancing the abrasion resistance, but retaining the mechanical properties.

In any case, both techniques require a subsequent thermal treatment close to or above the melting temperature, in order to eliminate the residual macroradical.

The differences in the crosslinking process and in the thermal treatment give reason of the presence on the market of cross-linked polyethylenes with a wide range of chemical, physical and mechanical properties.

Table 1:

Comparison Among New Crosslinked Thermally-Stabilized Polyethylenes.

(The processing parameters shown in this table were compiled from various publications, and information provided by the manufacturers is subject to ongoing modification.)

Name and Manufacturer	Radiation Type and Dose	Thermal Stabilization	Final Final Sterilization	Total Crosslinking Dose and Type
Marathon™ DePuy, Inc.	γ radiation to 50 kGy at room temperature	Remelted at 155°C for 24 hours followed by annealing at 120°C for 24 h.	Gas plasma	50 kGy gamma
XLPE™ Smith & Nephew – Richards, Inc.	γ radiation to 100 kGy at room temperature	Remelted at 150°C for two hours	Ethylene oxide	100 kGy gamma
Longevity™ Zimmer, Inc.	Electron beam radiation to 100 kGy at room temperature	Remelted at 150°C for about six hours	Gas plasma	100 kGy electron beam
Durasul™ Sulzer, Inc.	Electron beam radiation to 95 kGy at 125 °C	Remelted at 150°C for about two hours	Ethylene oxide	95 kGy electron beam
Crossfire™ Stryker-Osteonics-Howmedica, Inc.	γ radiation to 75 kGy at room temperature	Annealed at about 120°C for a proprietary duration	Gamma at 25 to 35 kGy while packaged in nitrogen	100 to 110 kGy of gamma
Aeonian™ Kyocera, Inc.	γ radiation to 35 kGy at room temperature	Annealed at 110°C for ten hours	Gamma at 25 to 40 kGy while packaged in nitrogen	60 to 75 kGy of gamma

Limitation

Abrasion of polymers is a complex process, depending on the physico-chemical properties of both the polymer and the abrading material.

In the present case, the polymer is cross-linked UHMWPE and the abrading material can be either a metallic or a ceramic surface, which have different roughness, or even a third body with various shape and hardness, such as bone or cement fragments or phosphate and ossalate crystals from the synovial fluid. The increase in the molecular mass of UHMWPE causes an increase in the resistance to abrasion with smooth abrading material (£ 10 micron). On the contrary, with rough counterfaces, the focal parameter is the toughness of the abraded material, thus the energy required for tearing material off the surface. Since the toughness of a cross-linked UHMWPE is lower than that of the untreated one, its resistance to abrasion with a material of roughness higher than 10 microns will be lower than that of virgin UHMWPE.

Conclusion

The first clinical results of cross-linked polyethylene do not show a considerable improvement of performances. This evidence was quite predictable from the existing literature studies. A larger number of case studies is necessary in order to evaluate the objective performances of the new material in different clinical conditions.

References

1. McKellop, H.A.; Campbell, P., Park, S.H.; Schmalzried, T.P.; Grigoris, P.; Amstutz, H.C.; Sarmiento A: The origin of submicron polyethylene wear debris in total hip arthroplasty. Clin Orthop 311: 3-20, 1995
2. Costa, L.; Luda, M.P.; Trossarelli, L.; Brach del Prever, E.M.; Crova, M.; Gallinaro, P.: Oxidation in orthopaedic UHMWPE sterilized by gamma-radiation and ethylene oxide. Biomaterials, 19:659-, 1998.
3. Kurtz, S.M., Muratoglu, O.K.; Evans, M.; Edidin, A.A.: Advances in the processing, sterilization, and crosslinking of UHMWPE for total joint arthroplasty. Biomaterials, 20:1659-1688, 1999.
4. McKellop, H.; Shen, F.-W.; Lu., B.; Salovey, R.; Campbell, P.: The effect of sterilization method and other modifications on the wear resistance of acetabular cups of ultra-high molecular weight polyethylene. A hip simulator study. J. Bone and Joint Surgery, 82-A (12), 1708-1725, 2000
5. Fisher, J.; Reeves, E. A.; Isaac, G. H.; Saum, K. A.; and Sanford, W. M.: Comparison of the wear of aged and non-aged UHMWPE sterilized by gamma irradiation and by gas plasma. J. Mater. Sci. Mater. Med., 8:375-378, 1997.
6. Costa L. and Brach del Prever E.M. "UHMWPE for Arthroplasty" Edizione Minerva Medica Torino 2000.
7. Shen, F.-W.; McKellop, H.: Interaction of oxidation and crosslinking in gamma-irradiated ultra-high molecular weight polyethylene. J Biomedical Materials Research, 61:430-439, 2002.
8. McKellop, H.; Shen, F.-W.; Lu, B.; Campbell, P.; Salovey, R.: Development of an extremely wear resistant UHMW polyethylene for total hip replacements. J. Orthopaedic Research. 17 (2), 157-167, 1999
9. Muratoglu, O.K.; Bragdon, C.R.; O'Connor, D.O.; Jasty, M.; Harris, W.H.: A novel method of crosslinking UHMWPE to improve wear, reduce oxidation, and retain mechanical properties. J Arthroplasty, 16:149-160, 2001.
10. Saikko, V.; Calonius, O.; Keranen, J.: Wear of conventional and crosslinked UHMWPE acetabular cups against polished and roughened CoCr femoral heads in biaxial hip simulator. J Biomed Mater Res (Appl Biomater), 63:848-853, 2002.
11. Affatato, S.; Bordini, B.; Fagnano, C.; Taddei, P.; Tinti, A.; Toni, A.: Effects of the sterilization method on the wear of UHMWPE acetabular cups tested in a hip joint simulator. Biomaterials, 23:1439-1446, 2002.
12. Grobbelaar, C. J.; Plessis, T. A. D.; Marais, F.: The radiation improvement of polyethylene prostheses. J. Bone and Joint Surg., 60-B:370-374, 1978.
13. Grobbelaar, C.J.; Weber, F.A.; Spirakis, A.; et al.: Clinical experience with gamma irradiation-crosslinked polyethylene – A 14 to 20 year follow-up report. South African Bone and Joint Surgery, XI(3):140-147, 1999.
14. Oonishi, H.; Takayama, Y.; and Tsuji, E.: Improvement of polyethylene by irradiation in artificial joints. Radiat. Phys. Chem., 39:495-504, 1992.
15. Oonishi, H.; Saito, M.; Kadoya, Y.: Wear of high-dose gamma irradiated polyethylene in total hip replacement: Long term radiological evaluation. Trans Orthop Res Soc, p97, 1998.
16. Wroblewski, B.M.; Siney, P.D.; Fleming, P.A.: Low-friction arthroplasty of the hip using alumina ceramic and crosslinked polyethylene : A ten-year follow-up report. J Bone Joint Surg., 81-B:54-55, 1999.

3.5 Reducing Wear Using the Ceramic Surface on Oxidized Zirconium Heads

V. Good, K. Widding, D. Heuer and G. Hunter

Introduction

Wear-related complications remain a major cause of revisions following total hip arthroplasty. Oxide ceramic modular heads were introduced as an alternative to metallic cobalt-chromium (CoCr) heads because their surfaces are more abrasion-resistant and produce less friction, thereby reducing abrasive and adhesive wear of the opposing polyethylene[1]. The use of oxide ceramic heads can reduce wear by 25 to 50% [2-5]. Oxidized zirconium (OxZr) was introduced as a way to provide these advantages in wear performance without the risks associated with brittle fracture of monolithic ceramics[6]. Thermally driven oxygen diffusion transforms just the metallic zirconium alloy surface into a durable, stable, low-friction oxide[7-9]. Thus, OxZr provides the benefits of ceramic wear behavior along with the mechanical properties of metal[10, 11]. This study assessed the wear properties of OxZr and CoCr heads against highly crosslinked polyethylene (XPE) that was irradiated at 10 Mrad and melt-annealed, as well as non-crosslinked polyethylene (NPE) that was not irradiated.

Materials and Methods

The NPE and XPE acetabular liners (32 mm, Reflection™, Smith & Nephew) were made of GUR1050 ultra high molecular weight polyethylene (Poly-Hi Solidur, Ft. Wayne, IN) and terminally sterilized using ethylene oxide. Half of the OxZr (Oxinium®) and CoCr heads (32 mm, Smith & Nephew) were tested with smooth surfaces (out of the box) and the rest were pre-roughened by tumbling in alumina particles in order to simulate the abrasive conditions of some clincally retrieved heads[12-15]. Both R_a and R_{pm} were used to measure the surface roughness. The thickness of the OxZr ceramic surface was monitored periodically during testing. Two measurements were made at the apex of the head and four were made 45° from the apex using a Fourier Transform Infrared (FTIR) spectrometer (Nexus 470, Nicolet, Madison, WI).

Simulator testing was conducted on a 12 station physiological hip simulator (AMTI, Watertown, MA) at 1 Hz in 450 ml of 100% bovine serum per station. Three specimens were tested per condition with soak-controls for fluid absorption correction. All conditions were tested to at least 5 Mcycle, and the OxZr with XPE combinations were continued to 20 Mcycle. Loading curves alternated between ISO and Bergman every 0.1 Mcycle[16,17]. Gravimetric measurements of polyethylene wear were corrected for fluid absorption and then used to calculate linear rates of volumetric wear using the density of the ultra high molecular weight polyethylene ($0.93 \ g/cm^3$). The wear debris was characterized using techniques described previously[18]. Statistical significance was determined using analysis of variance.

Results

In comparison to the smooth heads (<0.04 µm R_a), the pre-roughened heads appeared hazy with multi-directional scratches. The measurements of R_a (0.17 ± 0.1 mm) and R_{pm} (2.6 ± 0.35 µm) on the roughened CoCr heads were similar to those of some retrieved heads [12-15]. They were also significantly greater (p<0.01) than the measurements of R_a (0.06 ± 0.01 µm) and R_{pm} (0.16 ± 0.03 µm) on the roughened OxZr heads.

For the XPE liners during the first 5 Mcycle of testing, the OxZr heads in both the smooth and roughened conditions produced no detectable volumetric wear. The CoCr heads produced no detectable XPE wear in the smooth condition, but roughened CoCr produced 15.4 ± 4.1 mm³/Mcycle of XPE wear (Fig. 1).

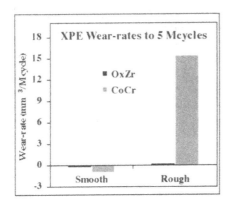

Figure 1:
Wear-rates of XPE articulating against OxZr and CoCr in both smooth and roughened conditions for a duration of 5 Mcycle.

Particle analysis of the XPE wear debris showed that significantly fewer particles (p=0.03) were produced by smooth OxZr heads (1.6 ± 0.8 million/cycle) than by smooth CoCr heads (2.2 ± 0.5 million/cycle). In the roughened condition, significantly fewer XPE particles (p<0.01) also were produced by OxZr (3.3 ± 1.2 million/cycle) than by CoCr (8.9 ± 3.3 million/cycle) heads (Fig. 2).

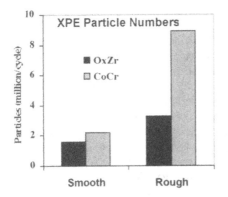

Figure 2:
Number of XPE particles generated when articulating against OxZr and CoCr in smooth and rough conditions for a duration of 5 Mcycle.

For the NPE liners during the first 5 Mcycle of testing, wear rates were significantly less (p<0.01) for smooth OxZr (21 ± 0.23 mm³/Mcycle) than for smooth CoCr (38 ± 0.58 mm³/Mcycle), and for roughened OxZr (30 ± 0.36 mm³/Mcycle) than for roughened CoCr (76 ± 3.8 mm³/Mcycle) heads (Fig. 3).

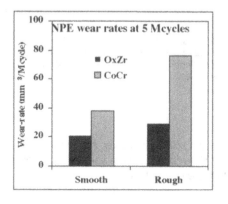

Figure 3:
Wear-rates of NPE articulating against OxZr and CoCr in both smooth and roughened conditions for a duration of 5 Mcycle.

Particle analysis of NPE wear debris showed that significantly fewer particles (p ≤ 0.01) were produced by smooth OxZr (5.6 ± 0.6 million/cycle) than smooth CoCr (8.0 ± 1.2 million/cycle), and by roughened OxZr (5.8 ± 0.6 million/cycle) than roughened CoCr (10.5 ± 3.0 million/cycle) heads (Fig. 4).

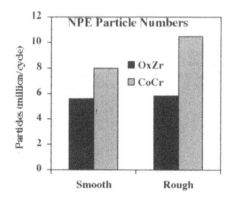

Figure 4:
Number of NPE particles generated when articulating against OxZr and CoCr in smooth and rough conditions for a duration of 5 Mcycle.

Tests with OxZr heads were continued on the simulator for another 15 Mcycle. The volumetric wear rate for XPE liners remained nondetectable with smooth OxZr heads, but by 20 Mcycle, the roughened OxZr heads produced a small amount (0.35 ± 0.04 mm³/Mcycle) of XPE wear (Fig. 5).

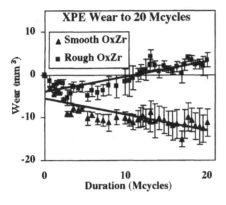

Figure 5:
Wear of XPE articulating against smooth and roughened OxZr heads for a duration of 20 Mcycle.

Measured changes in oxide thickness on the OxZr heads over the entire test duration were within the resolution of the FTIR technique, with linear regression indicating oxide wear rates of 0.0023 μm/Mcycle or less (Fig. 6).

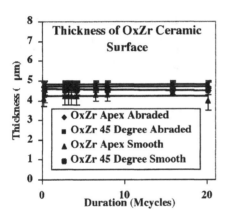

Figure 6:
OxZr ceramic surface thickness over 20 Mcycle of wear simulator testing.

Discussion

This study like previous studies has shown that XPE can provide substantial wear reductions compared to the performance of NPE [19, 20]. The volumetric wear reduction was significant when XPE was mated with a smooth CoCr surface; however, when the surface was roughened as is seen clinically with CoCr heads, the wear reduction was much less. Also important to note is that the roughened CoCr heads produced no statistical distinction (p=0.38) in the number of wear debris particles from the NPE and XPE liners. Conversely, the ceramic surface of the OxZr heads resisted roughening better than CoCr and helped maintain the superior XPE wear performance seen with smooth heads. This benefit also was demonstrated with NPE when mated with OxZr; volumetric wear rates were reduced by 45% and 61% when compared to CoCr under smooth and

Although volumetric wear of XPE couldn't be detected gravimetrically in some of these tests, it was clear that measurable wear debris was being produced. An estimation of XPE wear volume based on particle size and number was shown in a previous analysis to be approximately 1 mm³/Mcycle for smooth CoCr heads[21]. Using this same technique for smooth OxZr heads at 5 Mcycle, the volumetric wear rate of XPE is estimated to be 0.4 mm³/Mcycle. This indicates that OxZr produced approximately 60% less XPE wear than did CoCr. For smooth heads, it also indicates that XPE with OxZr produced about 98% less volumetric wear than was produced by NPE with CoCr.

Not only did the ceramic oxide surfaces of OxZr resist roughening better than the metallic surfaces of CoCr, but the loss of oxide thickness was negligible during the 20 Mcycle simulator tests even on the pre-roughened heads. This demonstrated the durability of the ceramic surface on the OxZr heads.

Conclusion

This study demonstrated the advantage of a low-friction and abrasion-resistant ceramic surface for articulation against polyethylene. Roughening the heads to a clinically relevant extent demonstrated that the durable oxide ceramic surfaces of OxZr heads can maintain the wear performance of crosslinked polyethylene better than the metallic surfaces of CoCr heads. These results suggest that the use of OxZr heads with XPE liners may contribute to reducing wear-related clincal complications.

References

1. Davidson JA (1993) Characteristics of metal and ceramic total hip bearing surfaces and their effect on long-term ultra high molecular weight polyethylene wear. Clin Orthop 294:361-378
2. Schmalzried TP, Scott DL, Zahiri, CA, Dorey FJ, Sanford WM, Kem L, Humphrey W (1998) Variables affecting wear in vivo: analysis of 1,080 hips with computer-assisted technique. Trans Orthop Res Soc 23:275
3. Sychterz CJ, Moon KH, Hashimoto AY, Terefenko KM, Engh CA, Bauer TW (1996) Wear of polyethylene cups in total hip arthroplasty a study of specimens retrieved post mortem. J Bone Joint Surg 78-A:1193-1200
4. Oonishi H, Takayaka Y, Clarke IC, Jung, H (1992) Comparative wear studies of 28-mm ceramic and stainless steel total hip joints over 2 to 7 year period. J Long-Term Effects Med Implants 2:37-47
5. Oonishi H, Kadoya Y (2000) Wear of high-dose gamma-irradiated polyethylene in total hip replacements. J Orthop Sci 5:223-228
6. Laskin RS (2003) An oxidized Zr ceramic surfaced femoral component for total knee arthroplasty. Clin Orthop 416:191-196
7. Benezra V, Mangin S, Treska M, Spector M, Hunter G, Hobbs LW (1999) Microstructural investigation of the oxide scale on Zr-2.5Nb and its interface with the alloy substrate. In: Neenan T, Marcolongo M, Valentini RF (eds) Biomedical Materials. Materials Research Society, Warrendale, PA, Symp Proc 550, pp 337-342
8. Hunter G, Long M (2000) Abrasive wear of oxidized Zr-2.5Nb, CoCrMo, and Ti-6Al-4V against bone cement. Trans Sixth World Biomater Cong: 835
9. Hunter G (2001) Adhesion testing of oxidized zirconium. Trans Soc Biomater 24:540

10. Sprague J, Aldinger P, Tsai S, Hunter G, Thomas R, Salehi A (2003) Mechanical behavior of zirconia, alumina, and oxidized zirconium modular heads. In: Brown S, Clarke IC, Gustafson A (eds) ISTA 2003. International Society for Technology in Arthroplasty, Birmingham, AL, vol 2: in press

11. Tsai S, Spargue J, Hunter G, Thomas R, Salehi A (2001) Mechanical testing and finite element analysis of oxidized zirconium femoral components. Trans Soc Biomater 24:163

12. Barrack RL, Castro FP, Szuszczewicz ES, Schmalzried TP (2002) Analysis of retrieved uncemented porous-coated acetabular components in patients with and without pelvic osteolysis. Orthopedics 25:1373-1378

13. Ries M, Salehi A, Widding K, Hunter G (2002) Polyethylene wear performance of oxidized zirconium and cobalt-chromium knee components under abrasive conditions. J Bone Joint Surg 84-A(S2):129-135

14. Hall RM, Siney P, Unsworth A, Wroblewski BM (1997) The effect of surface topography of retrieved femoral on the wear of UHMWPE sockets. Med Eng Phys 19:711-719

15. Jasty M, Bragdon CR, Lee K, Hanson A, Harris WH (1994) Surface damage to cobalt-chrome femoral head prostheses. J Bone Joint Surg 76-B:73-77

16. ISO/DIS 14242-1: 1999-06 (1997) Implants for surgery – wear of total hip-joint prostheses – Part 1: loading and displacement parameters for wear-testing machines and corresponding environmental conditions for test. International Organization for Standardization, Geneva

17. Bergmann G, Graichein F, Rohlmann A (1993) Hip joint loading during walking and running, measured in two patients. J Biomech 26:969-990

18. Ries MD, Scott ML, Shilesh J (2001) Relationship between gravimetric wear and particle generation in hip simulators: conventional compared with cross-linked polyethylene. J Bone Joint Surg 83-A(S2):116-122

19. Furman BD, Bhattacharyya S, Hernoux C, Ranawat CS, Li S (2001) Independent evaluation of wear properties of commercially available cross linked UHMWPE. Trans Soc Biomater 24:33

20. Greenwald AS, Bauer TW, Ries, MD (2001) New poly for old: contribution or caveat? J Bone Joint Surg 83-A(S2):27-31

21. Morrison M, Scott M, Mishra SR, Jani S (2002) Determination of UHMWPE wear particle volume using atomic force microscopy. Trans Soc Biomater 25:296

3.6 Is the OXINIUM Technology a Useful Technology in Total Joint Arthroplasty?

C. B. Rieker

What is the OXINIUM Technology?

The OXINIUM technology, developed by Smith & Nephew, is designed to oxidize a wrought 97.5% zirconium – 2.5% niobium alloy by means of thermal diffusion and so create a zirconia surface about 5 µm thick [1], as shown in Figure 1 [1].

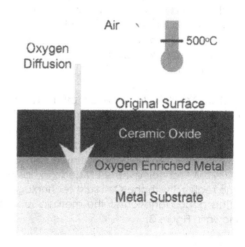

Figure 1:
The OXINIUM technology.

This zirconia layer on the zirconium-niobium alloy is not an externally applied coating, but the original metal transformed into zirconium-oxide ceramic.

According to the information published by Smith & Nephew [2] and shown in Figure 2, the nano-hardness of the zirconia layer ranges from 14 – 15 GPa. This nano-hardness is much higher than that of the untreated alloy, which is about 3 GPa. An abrupt hardness transition is evident at the interface, i.e. between the ceramic oxide and the oxygen-enriched metal. This confirms that the surface treatment of the zirconium-niobium alloy may have the same behaviour as a coating. Such an abrupt hardness transition may involve the risk of sub-surface interface cracking due to internal stresses, and could lead to the delamination of the zirconia layer.

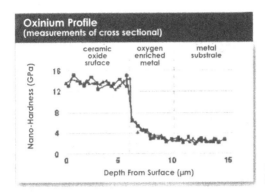

Figure 2:
Nano-hardness profile.

The information published by Smith & Nephew [3] states that all the tests performed during the development stage (abrasive wear tests, adhesive wear tests, friction tests against cartilage, oxide adhesion tests, fatigue tests, hip simulator tests, knee simulator tests, biocompatibility tests) were completed positively. The OXINIUM technology is therefore available for both total hip and knee prostheses.

This OXINIUM technology offers an advanced surface with good wear properties. These properties are definitively better than those of the underlying zirconium-niobium alloy. Hence, should the layer fail for any particular reason, the tribologic situation may lead to a large amount of metallic wear.
Such failures are well documented with TiN coatings on titanium alloys. Like the OXINIUM technology, the TiN coating has a high hardness (even higher than the one realized with the OXINIUM technology), a thickness of about 5 µm and also offers good adhesion to the metallic substrate. An example of such a failure is shown in Figure 3.

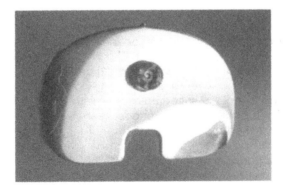

Figure 3:
Failure of a TiN coating.

The TiN coating on the tibial baseplate of this mobile bearing, total knee prosthesis, failed after an implantation time of only 7 months.

OXINIUM Technology for Total Hip Prostheses

According to Smith & Nephew [2] and also V. Good et al. [4], the OXINIUM technology offers the following advantages for total hip prostheses:
- Lower polyethylene wear rate in comparison with CoCr ball heads.
  Wear reduction of 98% in combination with highly cross-linked polyethylene.
- Lower production of polyethylene wear particles.
- Due to the higher hardness, the OXINIUM ball heads offer better resistance to scratches than CoCr ball heads.
- No risk of fracture with OXINIUM ball heads.

These advantages are well documented.

However, similar results may be obtained by using other technologies:
- Even higher wear rate reductions have been measured by different laboratories using conventional CoCr ball heads and highly cross-linked polyethylenes [5]. These spectacular wear reductions, which are due to the extreme wear resistance of the newly developed highly cross-linked polyethylenes, are hardly influenced by the OXINIUM technology.
- A recent review of the literature by Dumbleton et al. [6] has shown that osteolysis is rarely observed when the polyethylene wear rate is less than 0.1 mm/y. The authors suggest that a practical wear-rate threshold of 0.05 mm/y would eliminate osteolysis. Since such wear rates were measured in-vitro with highly cross-linked polyethylenes, this review implies that highly cross-linked polyethylenes would eliminate osteolysis. In such a case, the lower production of wear particles observed in-vitro with the OXINIUM ball heads has no clinical relevance.
- Plain ceramic ball heads (alumina heads, zirconia heads and zirconia-toughened alumina heads) have a comparable or an even higher hardness than the OXINIUM ball heads. Furthermore, they offer the same or even better resistance against scratches than OXINIUM ball heads.
- Being a metallic ball head with a zirconia layer on its surface, the OXINIUM ball head cannot fracture like an alumina or zirconia head. A similar fracture resistance has also been observed with newly developed and tougher ceramic materials (for example, zirconia-toughened alumina) and has not resulted in any in-vivo fracture to date [7].

OXINIUM Technology for Total Knee Prostheses

According to M. Spector et al. [1], Smith & Nephew [2] and M. Ries et al. [8], the OXINIUM technology offers the following advantages for total knee prostheses:
- Lower polyethylene wear rate in comparison with a CoCr femoral component - wear reduction of 85%.
- Lower polyethylene wear rate in comparison with a CoCr femoral component in the abraded condition – eight-fold wear reduction.
- Lower production of polyethylene wear particles.

These advantages are well documented.

These better wear properties of OXINIUM femoral components are certainly interesting, but do not solve one of the major tribologic problems of total knee prostheses, namely the delamination of the polyethylene insert [9]. This is attributable to the synergical effects that result from the mechanical overloading of the polyethylene (contact stresses in excess of 20 MPa) and an in-vivo oxidation of the polyethylene. The following strategies will have to be implemented to reduce the incidence of delamination:

- Better congruency will have to be designed between the articulating surfaces. This will increase the areas of contact and lower the stress sustained by the polyethylene. Modern knee designs (fixed bearing or mobile bearing total knee prostheses) are an efficient way of improving the matching of the articulating surfaces.
- A highly cross-linked polyethylene without free radicals is the best available method [5] for minimizing the in-vivo oxidation of the polyethylene.

When these two strategies are combined, the probability of delamination is kept very low and independent of the material used to manufacture the femoral component (OXINIUM technology or conventional CoCr alloy).

Furthermore, the abrasive/adhesive polyethylene wear rate observed in-vitro in total knee prostheses is much lower than that observed in-vitro in total hip prostheses. For example, the following wear rates were published in the OXINIUM studies:

- CoCr femoral component [8] for knee: 4.7 ± 2.3 mm^3/10^6 cycles
- CoCr femoral component [4] for hip: 38 ± 0.6 mm^3/10^6 cycles

The observed wear rate for total knee prostheses is eight times less than that observed by hip prostheses and such a low wear rate could be below the threshold level for osteolysis.

Discussion

The OXINIUM technology is an elegant technology for adding a zirconia layer to a zirconium-niobium alloy.

Being a hard layer on a soft metallic substrate, the interface between the ceramic oxide and the oxygen-enriched metal has to be carefully manufactured to avoid any risk of delamination. Furthermore, should the layer fail, the tribologic situation may lead to a large amount of metallic wear, which has been the case with TiN coatings.

There are alternative-bearing systems with similar or better wear properties for total hip prostheses. Most of these systems have been clinically approved and do not entail the risks induced by any new technology.

The OXINIUM technology does not help to solve the main tribologic problem that has to be met with total knee prostheses – the delamination of the polyethylene insert.

Being a new technology, the OXINIUM was tested extensively in-vitro (abrasive wear tests, adhesive wear tests, friction tests against cartilage, oxide adhesion tests, fatigue tests, hip simulator tests, knee simulator tests, biocompatibility tests) prior to its market launch. As these tests provided positive results, the OXINIUM technology was made progressively available to the orthopaedic community. For a new technology like the OXINIUM, it is extremely difficult to estimate all the tests to be conducted and to determine the severity of these tests. And even with a comprehensive test program, it is not possible to obtain the 100% confidence that the in-vivo behaviour will match up with the in-vitro results. For instance, the interface of OXINIUM uncemented components with the bone substrate is extremely difficult to investigate in-vitro.

Smith & Nephew may have experienced such difficulties with the OXINIUM technology, because the sale of two uncemented OXINIUM femoral components (GENESIS II and PROFIX) was stopped in September 2003. According to the available information, about 1% of these uncemented femoral OXINIUM components became loose. Unfortunately, Smith & Nephew has not released any further information on this matter.

Conclusions

The OXINIUM technology is a sophisticated technology for covering a zirconium-niobium alloy with a thin zirconia layer. Due to its higher hardness, this technology helps to lower the amount of adhesive/abrasive polyethylene wear observed on total joint prostheses.

Like any new technology released in the field of orthopaedics, the technology has to be monitored carefully before its propagation on a large scale. Since some of the unexplained problems seem to have been caused by two types of OXINIUM femoral component, I would not recommend the use of this OXINIUM technology before a clear explanation of these events is forthcoming. Furthermore, alternative solutions with greater clinical experience than the OXINIUM technology are available for reducing the adhesive/abrasive polyethylene wear rate observed in total hip and knee arthroplasties.

References

1. Spector M., et al.; Wear performance of UHMWPE on oxidized zirconium total knee femoral components; The Journal of Bone and Joint Surgery – Supplement 2, part 2, 2001, 83A, p. 80.
2. http://www.oxidizedzirconium.com/2100_oxmaterial.html; downloaded on February 4, 2004.
3. http://www.oxidizedzirconium.com/default.html; downloaded on February 10, 2004.
4. Good V., et al.; Reduced wear with oxidized zirconium femoral heads; The Journal of Bone and Joint Surgery – Supplement 4, 2003, 85A, p. 105.
5. Muratoglu O.K., Bragdon C.R., O'Connor D.O., Jasty M., Harris W.H.; A novel method of cross-linking ultra-high-molecular-weight polyethylene to improve wear, reduce oxidation, and retain mechanical properties; Journal of Arthroplasty, 2001, 16, p. 149.
6. Dumbleton J.H., Manley M.T., Edidin A.A.; A literature review of the association between wear rate and osteolysis in total hip arthroplasty; Journal of Arthroplasty, 2002, 17, p. 649.
7. Willmann G., Personal communication; February 12, 2004.

8. Ries M., et al.; Polyethylene wear performance of oxidized zirconium and cobalt-chrome knee components under abrasive conditions; The Journal of Bone and Joint Surgery – Supplement 2, 2002, 84A, p. 129.
9. Bohl J.R., Bohl W.R., Postak P.D., Greenwald A.S.; The effects of shelf life on clinical outcome for gamma sterilized polyethylene tibial components; Clin. Orthop. 1999, 367, p. 28.

3.7 Ceramic Coatings in Metal-PE Joints: Where Are We Now?

C. Piconi, G. Maccauro and F. Muratori

Abstract

Several types of hard coatings were applied onto metallic components in arthroprostheses' bearings to reduce UHMWPE wear and the consequent wear debris-induced periprosthetic osteolysis, that is still the main problem in arthroplasty. This approach was aimed to obtain in the surface of metal components finish and scratch resistance similar to the ones of alumina ceramic components. Many attempts were made to improve the surface properties of stainless steel, of cobalt-chromium, of titanium alloys and of zirconium alloys. Arthroprostheses' bearing components coated by titanium nitride (TiN) or diamond-like carbon (DLC), and more recently zirconium-2,5 Nb alloy with a surface layer of monoclinic zirconium dioxide were introduced on the market. This paper briefly reviews the literature on ceramic coatings in prosthetic bearings to assess the today's status of this technology in arthroplasty.

Introduction

Metal-on-polyethylene bearings are still the most used in arthroplasty [1], performing with satisfactory outcomes especially in older, less active patients [2]. From a long time polyethylene was identified as the main source of debris-induced periprosthetic osteolysis that is still among the main causes of implants failure. Many attempts made to reduce the wear of metal-on-polyethylene bearings, focussed on both components of the joint. Research was addressed both to improve the tribological properties of polyethylene e.g. by introduction of second phases or by enhancing the polymeric chains cross-linking, both to improve by a ceramic coating the hardness and the finish stability of metallic THR ball heads and femoral TKR components. The results achieved on the latter topic are briefly reviewed in the following.

Physical Vapor Deposition (PVD) Coatings

Plasma spray coatings are not of help in bearings, due to their limits in adhesion to the substrate and to their residual porosity. The most commonly used processes Physical Vapor Deposition (PVD) technologies, e.g. Arc Vapor Deposition, Sputtering (Magnetron Sputtering) and Electron Beam evaporation. Briefly, PVD process consists in the generation of a plasma of metal ions that are "transported" by an electric field to the surface to be coated. Depending on the process, the behaviour of the plasma may be different, obtaining in turn coatings with different properties notwithstanding the same name. The common characteristics of these processes is that the parts to be coated must be exposed to the plasma, and are then referred as "line of sight" processes. This fact may have significant implication when complex shapes are to be coated, like e.g. in the case of the femoral component of knee replacements.

Titanium Nitride Coatings

TiN is a popular wear protective coating so far, and is used also for its brilliant golden colour to improve the aspect of objects like e.g. door handles. Being biocompatible [3], TiN coatings are used also in several biomedical applications, including dental instruments, dentures, orthodontic archwires, endovascular stents and catheters.

TiN coatings may show very high internal stresses due to differences in coating properties at local level depending on the deposition process parameters (e.g. reaction environment, presence of impurities, rate of formation, angle of deposition), that joined to the relatively low adhesion may lead to the spallation of the coating from the substrate. The use of higher coating temperatures, that lead to some diffusion bonding, or of an interlayer may improve the coating characteristics. TiN coatings were applied in hip, knee, ankle and shoulder replacements, but little exists in the literature concerning their clinical outcomes. Positive clinical results after ten years of a series of 50 TiN coated total ankle replacements was recently reported [4], but other reports are raising concerns about the ability of TiN coatings to withstand wear damage in clinical applications [5] and the analysis of THR heads retrieved after clinical use [6] put in evidence extensive abrasion of the coating, that reached about 70% of the articulating surface in the case of an high-demand heavy patient.

Diamond-Like Carbon Coatings

The name of Diamond-Like Carbon (DLC) identifies a class of carbon-based materials, characterised by the simultaneous presence of sp^3 and sp^2 C-C chemical bonds giving them structure and properties intermediate between diamond and graphite. The characteristics of these materials are often described by the ratio sp^3/sp^2, e.g. the concentration of diamond-type bonds vs. the graphite ones, which value is depending on deposition conditions of the film. The structure of DLC films, that may be described as a dispersion of diamond "nodules" in a graphite matrix, is inherently metastable, and may transform to graphite at high temperatures or under irradiation. Also in DLC coatings the main problem is the adhesion to the substrate, as the interfacial residual stresses may reach very high values within the 1-2 μm thick coating layer.

The biocompatibility of DLC coatings is a well documented behaviour [7,8] and was confirmed also by recent studies [9]. Notwithstanding the fact that it is known at least DLC coated ball heads are in clinical use the literature is concerning only laboratory tests, that gave controversial results. Wear tests aimed to evaluate DLC as a coating for tibial trays of knee prostheses [10] measured 3.5 increase in wear of UHMWPE pins sliding against DLC-coated Vs. cast CoCr alloy plates, leading the Authors to remark the unsuitability of DLC coating for the intended application. Also the results of biaxial hip simulator tests were controversial: similar wear of UHMWPE cups against CoCr DLC-coated and uncoated heads was reported [11], both values higher than the wear of the same cups against alumina heads, while other Authors [12] measured wear rates of UHMWPE cups similar for Alumina and DLC coated heads, both higher than CoCr coupled to the same cups. In pin-on-disk tests against PMMA pins [13] DLC coated Ti6Al4V disks performed worse than wrought CoCrMo alloy raising doubts about coating resistance to third body wear.

An original bearing couple DLC-on-DLC was tested in a simplified hip simulator and in pin-on-disk wear tests with satisfactory results [14], but this bearing couple was not transferred to clinic up to now.

In-Situ Zirconia Coating

The formation of hard zirconium dioxide (ZrO_2) layer on zirconium alloys to protect them from corrosion is a very well known process, used in the past to protect the claddings of Zircalloy-2 nuclear fuel pins from fretting corrosion on spacer grids in Light Water Reactors [15]. Black or blue-black zirconium dioxide layers may be obtained on zirconium alloys in air, in steam or in water at temperature between 350 and 600°C [16], or in molten salts like chlorides, nitrates, cyanides at temperatures in the range 700-800°C [17].

Composition		Mechanical Properties	
Zr	Min 95,5	Density (g/cm³)	6,44
Fe+Cr	0,2	Yeld Strength (MPa)	380
Hf	Max 4,5	U.T.S. (MPa)	552
Nb	2,5	Fracture Strain (%)	16
O	0,18	Young Modulus (GPa)	98

Microindentation tests [18] put in evidence that the oxide layer formed in-situ increase the hardness to about 14 GPa for a depth some 5 µm beneath the surface, then in 3-4 µm the hardness drops to the value of the underlying zirconium alloy (about 3 GPa).

Oxidised zirconium gave positive results in laboratory tests. Pin-on-disk wear tests against cartilage pins allowed to assess its suitability for emiarthroplasty [19], and tests against PMMA pins assessed the effectiveness of the treatment in protecting the soft metallic zirconium alloy against scratching due to third bodies in the joint [13]. Similar positive results were reported in knee simulator tests performed on femoral components in comparison with CoCr [20]. Further knee simulator tests showed a remarkable reduction in wear rate of UHMWPE tibial inserts running against oxidized zirconium alloy in comparison with CoCr alloy, the reported wear rates were 4,68 mm³/Million cycles against and 0,69 mm³/Million cycles, respectively [21]. The treatment proven its effectiveness also in THR ball heads: UHMWPE-oxidized zirconium alloy couple showed in hip simulator tests a significant reduction in wear in comparison to UHMWPE -CoCr alloy couple both in clean, both in abrasive wear conditions [22].

Discussion and Conclusions

Ceramic coating perform very well in reducing wear and friction in engineering applications, and then their application on metallic components of arthroprostheses to reduce UHMWPE wear appeared a attractive to solve the problem of debris-induced periprosthetic osteolysis. The analysis of the literature shows that the significant research effort devoted to develop TiN and DCL coatings for artroprostheses' bearings by many research groups worldwide has not led to widespread clinical applications up to now. On the other hand, oxidised zirconium layers formed by in-situ reaction on zirconium alloy looks very promising.

Laboratory wear tests of UHMWPE coupled to TiN coated metals are rather controversial, and joined to the reports of cases of TiN coating delamination [5,6] may have decreased the interest for the use this coating in arthroprostheses. Also the laboratory tests on DLC coatings show controversial results on the improvements in wear achieved by this treatment in comparison to CoCr alloy. Research aimed to control by optimised deposition conditions the high internal stresses of these extremely thin coatings to avoid coating spallation and detachment are still in progress.

Oxidised zirconium layers were reported to reduce PE wear with respect to CoCr alloy both in simulated hip and knee bearing conditions [21,22], and on these basis positive clinical outcomes may be expected. The recent voluntary withdrawal from the market of uncemented oxidised zirconium knees due to some early loosening [23] seems unrelated to the wear behaviour of the coating. While a significant mass of data about laboratory tests on ceramic coatings is present in the literature, at the best of author's knowledge only one report concerning the clinical outcomes of ceramic coatings on metallic bearing surfaces of arthroprostheses was published up to now, concerning TiN-coated ankle replacements [4]. The lack of reports of clinical results on ceramic coatings applied on arthroprosthes bearings was on already remarked by Sauer and Antony [1] in their 1998 review, and the same situation may be remarked today: notwithstanding the time elapsed and the progresses made the literature is still concerning laboratory tests only.

References

1. Sauer WL, Antony ME Predicting the clinical wear performance of orthopedic bearing surface. In: Jacobs JJ, Craig TL, eds, Alternative bearing surfaces in total joint replacements (ASTM-STP 1346), ASTM Publ, 1998 West Conshohocken, PA, USA, pp. 1-29.
2. Black J. Prospects for alternate bearing surfaces in total replacement arthroplasty of the hip. In: Puhl W, ed, Performance of the wear couple BIOLOX forte in hip arthroplasty, Enke publ, 1997 Stuttgart, Germany, pp. 2-10.
3. Paschoal AL, Vanadio EC, De Campos Franceschini Canale L, Lopes da Silva O, Huerta-Vilca D, de Jesus Montheo A. Metallic biomaterials TiN coated: corrosion analysis and biocompatibility. Artif Org 2003;27: 461-464.
4. Buechel FF sr, Buechel FF jr, Pappas MJ. Ten years evaluation of cementless Buechel-Peppas meniscal bearing total ankle replacemet. Foot Ankle Int 2003;24:462-72.
5. Harman MK, Banks SA, Hodge WA. Wear analysis of a retrieved hip implant with titanium nitride coating. J Arthroplasty 1997;12:938-45.

6. Raimondi MT, Pietrabissa R. The in-vivo wear performance of prosthetic femoral heads with titanium nitride coating. Biomaterials 2000;21: 907-13.

7. Thompson LA, Law FC, Rushton N, Franks J. Biocompatibility of diamond-like carbon coatings. Biomaterials 1991;12:37-40.

8. Parker TL, Parker KL, McColl IR, Grant DM, Wood JV. The biocompatibility of low temperature diamond-like carbon films: a transmission electron microscopy, scanning electron microscopy and cytotoxicity study. Diamond Rel Mater 1994;3:1120-23.

9. Allen M, Myer B, Rushton N. In-vivo and in-vitro investigations in the biocompatibility of diamond-like carbon (DLC) coatings for orthopedic applications. J Biomed Mater Res:Appl Biomater 2001;58:319-28.

10. Jones VC, Barton DC, Auger DD, Hardacker C, Stone MH, Fischer J. Simulation of tibial counterface wear in mobile bearing knees with uncoated and ADLC coated surfaces. Biomed Mater Eng 2001;11:105-15.

11. Saikko V, Ahlroos T, Calonius O, Keränen J. Wear simulation of total hip prostheses with polyethylene against CoCr, alumina and diamond-like carbon. Biomaterials 2001;22: 1507-14.

12. Affatato S, Frigo M, Toni A. An in vitro investigation of diamond-like carbon as a femoral head coating. J Biomed Mater Res: Appl Biomater 2000;53:221-26.

13. Mishra AK, Davidson JA. Abrasion Resistance of candidate coatings for orthopedic articulating surfaces. In: Doherty PJ, et al, eds, Advances in Biomaterials 10, Elsevier Science publ, 1992 Amsterdam, NL: 111-21.

14. Lappainen R, Anttila A, Heinonen H. Diamond coated Total Hip replacements. Clin Orthop 1998;352:118-27.

15. Conte M, Borello A, Cabrini N. (1976) Anodic oxidation of Zircalloy-2. J Appl Elettrochem 1976;6:293-99.

16. Watson (1961) US Patent 2,987,352.

17. Haygarth JC (1987) US Patent 4,671,824.

18. Long M, Riester L, Hunter GB. Proc. 24th SFB, 1998San Diego, CA, USA: 528.

19. Patel AM, Spector M. Tribological evaluation of oxidized zirconium using an articular cartilage counterface: a novel material for potential use in hemiarthroplasty. Biomaterials 1997;18:441-47.

20. White SE, Whiteside LA, McCarthy DS, Antony M, Poggie RA. Simulated knee wear with cobalt chromium and oxidized zirconium knee femoral components. Clin Orthop 1994;309:176-84.

21. Spector M, Ries MD, Bourne R, Sauer W, Long M, Hunter GB. UHMWPE wear performance of oxidized zirconium total knee femoral components. 68Th AAOS, 2001 San Francisco, CA, USA, Scientific Exhibit SE034.

22. Good V, Ries MD, Barrack RL, Widding K, Hunter GB, Heuer D. (2003) Reduced wear with oxidized zirconium femoral heads. 70th AAOS, New Orleans, LA, USA, Scientific Exhibit SE 213.

23. Gibbs G. Knee implant recall hits Smith & Nephew. The Guardian (UK), September 18 2003.

3.8 Metal on Metal in Resurfacing Arthroplasty: Risks or Benefits?

M. Menge

Introduction

At the beginning of hip endoprosthetics was the substitution of destroyed cartilage by biologigal or artificial materials. However, successful results were only achieved after the introduction of abrasion-resistant materials in combination with exactly matching differences of diameter (radial clearance) of head and socket. The cobalt-based alloy Vitallium® which had been introduced into medical therapy by dentists in 1932 was used by Smith-Petersen [1, 2] to create the world's first hemiprosthesis (1937) available on the market. The first total hip replacement was implanted by Wiles in London, who used a metal on metal joint made of stainless steel. In the course of the development of arthroplasty and after the introduction of bone cement, the successful period of THR began. Despite the excellent long-term results achieved for metal on metal prostheses (McKee-Farrar [10], Ring) which have been implanted since the sixties, hard on soft material configurations as specified by Charnley for his Low Friction Arthroplasty have been used at an increasing extent since the mid-seventies. The reasons for this were the excellent initial results obtained from the use of such prostheses. Apart from that, abrasion and loosening of acetabular cups due to equatorial jamming had occurred in some metal on metal prostheses in which the radial clearance provided for had been inappropriate. Moreover, there had been doubts in respect of possible allergic reactions and the possibility of carcinogenic effects of the metal particles at that time already [1]. The triumphant clinical advance of THRs using metal femoral heads and plastic acetabular cups continued until the problem of polyethylene abrasion and the destruction of bone induced by particle debris occurred and required new approaches to be developed [5]. This "particle disease" stopped, either, new attempts of resurfacing arthroplasty using a metal cap which was placed on the preserved bone of the femoral head, and a thin polyethylene cup, which had been rediscovered by Wagner and other authors.

For reintroduction of the metal on metal prostheses in 1988, the long-term results observed for McKee-Farrar and Ring prostheses which meanwhile had been published were referred to [10]. Weber propagated the use of a modular component system consisting of a 28mm femoral head and a corresponding metal cup [18], and after more than 150,000 implantations which had been carried out worldwide in more than 15 years it can be stated that the theoretical fears in respect of allergic or malignant effects have not been confirmed [4]. McMinn [12] caused the total resurfacing arthroplasty to be developed further and introduced it into clinical application as metal on metal bearing in 1991 (fig. 1 and 2). The results obtained seem to confirm his theory: the clinical results obtained have been excellent, the implant-specific risk is low, luxation safety is much higher than with smaller femoral heads, and there haven't been any side effects caused by stress shielding observed for resurfacing prostheses compared to stem-type prostheses. The preservation of the joint's natural biomechanics and

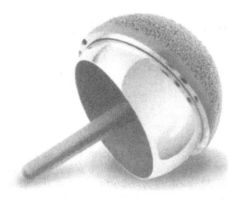

Figure 1:
Resurfacing prosthesis acc. to McMinn
(picture supplied by manufacturer).

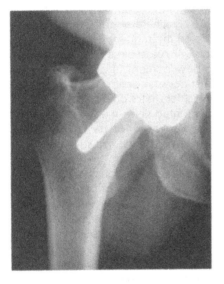

Figure 2:
Radiograph of a resurfacing prosthesis acc.
to McMinn.

the proprioceptive functions of the proximal femur make this implant particularly suited for active patients [12, 13]. Apart from that, the resurfacing prosthesis according to McMinn and the variants thereof stand out for their comparably good reviseability in case of failure of the implantation.

Design conditions to be complied with by resurfacing prostheses

There are high demands placed on the structural design of double-cup prostheses: only materials featuring high hardness and resistance to abrasion must be used, and the production process must guarantee a high degree of sphericity including specified radial clearances for polar high conformity load transition. In this respect, the bioinert alumina-based ceramics would be suited perfectly. Wagner had used a ceramic femoral head before (fig. 3), but so far it has not been possible to manufacture suitable cups with corresponding rear surface design to enable the cup's integration into the acetabulum as was stated by leading ceramics manufacturers.

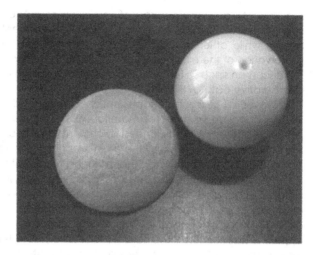

Figure 3:
Explanted resurfacing
prosthesis acc. to Wagner
with ceramic component.

The use of cobalt-based alloys with a carbide content of more than 3% ensures low surface wear under the geometric conditions mentioned above [3]. The relatively low speed of motion of the corresponding implant surfaces will not allow for reliable lubricating fluid-films to establish on the hydrophobe metal surfaces, and hence strain-related metal abrasion especially in the run-in phase cannot be eliminated.

Resurfacing prostheses are made of a cobalt-based alloy (residual), chromium (26.5 – 30%), molybdenum (4.5 – 7.0%), nickel (2.5%) and minor quantities of iron (<1%), manganese (<1%) and silicon (<1%), and in addition contain carbon at a rate of approx. 0.25 - 0.35% to enhance the material's hardness (alloy type HS 21). After the casting process, hard block carbides consisting of molybdenum, chromium and carbon are produced during congelation as a result of the carbon content, the total formula of which is $M_{23}C_6$ (fig. 4 from [15]). Although it is possible to enhance the material's strength by way of secondary thermal treatment and/or forging processes, this will also cause changes in the structure of the carbides (more refined distribution, smaller grain size of different structure (M_7C_3)).

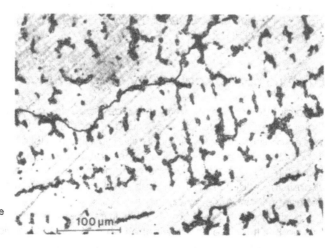

Figure 4:
"As cast" surface structure
of the cast alloy HS21
from [15].

The majority of manufacturers of metal on metal resurfacing prostheses use strength-enhancing processes such as solution treatment, hot isostatic pressing or forging while others restrain from any kind of heat treatment for the sake of preservation of the block carbides [12, 16]. The author shall not go into detail on this discussion since so far there haven't been sufficient quantities of independent comparative data available.

However, all of the products mentioned before have one thing in common: fretting corrosion and loss of material will be incurred especially in the run-in phase as a result of insufficient establishment of lubricating fluid films. As a result, the carbide peaks break and the grain tear out will be available in the organism as abrasion particles (fretting). The material's high resistance to abrasion will then be ensured by the flattened block carbides which are located slightly above the surface. The quantity of metal particles is determined either as abrasion thickness or by way of volumetric measurement. For Metasul[R] for instance, an abrasion rate of 25 µm/year is reported by the manufacturer for the run-in phase, and of approx. 5 µm/year for the time after the run-in phase [4] (values determined by way of simulator testing), whereas an abrasion rate of approx. 3 to 6 µm/year is indicated for the large surfaces of resurfacing prostheses for which correspondingly higher speeds of motion are incurred and hence the establishment of lubricating films is improved [3]. In the run-in phase, a temporary "squeaking noise" is sometimes reported by the patients for instance when they climb up stairs slowly. In the aggressive body environment, abrasion is subject to chemical reactions (contact corrosion) as far as there is no possibility of repassivation of the surfaces.

Hence the cobalt and chromium levels in the blood are especially high during the run-in phase but also later on depending on the strain level. Jacobs [8] reported an increase of the chromium level in the serum by factor 9, while the cobalt level ranged below the detection limit. The cobalt and chromium levels available in the whole blood after implantation of 28 mm metal femoral heads in combination with corresponding metal cups were investigated by Lhotka et al. [9] who in the follow-up examinations found that the blood levels of both metals were increased significantly by up to factor 10, with the whole-blood examinations also considering the particles stored in the intracellular space.

However, one of the substantial demands placed on implants is that "the tissue and organs of the implant recipient must not be damaged in any way by either the implant material as such, nor by any particles which may be released from it" (Ungethüm 1984 [15]).

Potential hazards caused by metal abrasion

Carcinogenic effects have been detected for a multitude of substances. Tumours were for instance provoqued in rodents by the implantation of solid bodies or dust particles of gold, silver, platinum, nickel, titanium and also of cobalt-based alloys [7,11]. Since the carcinogenic effect of cobalt and of chromium as a result of vapour inhalation has been detected in man, the undesirable side effects of such implant materials have been discussed permanently since the sixties.

Cobalt is considered an essential trace element and is also contained in vitamin B_{12}. It is stored mainly in the liver and discharged via the kidneys or the intestines. Nutritional over dosage has been observed in beer drinkers and was found to cause cardiomyopathy. Hence the use of cobalt salts as foam stabilizers in beer production was prohibited. There hasn't been any carcinogenic effect detected as a result of oral uptake of cobalt compounds. So far, it has not been possible to define any limits for cobalt levels in the blood for reasons of the data available [6, 7].

Natural chromium compounds usually are trivalent and do not have any significant biological effect. The hexavalent chromium compounds seem to be much more questionable but usually are observed in connection with technical production processes only (metal vapours in foundries). Intoxications are extremely rare. In the animal experiments, mutagenic effects were detected as a result of administration of hexavalent chromium salts [6, 7]. However, any possible oxidation processes of chromium-containing corrosion particles in the body will involve the relatively harmless trivalent compounds only.

Nickel was found to provoque malignant tumours in rodents as a result of parenteral administration. Such effect has not been observed for alloys with low nickel content [7]. There aren't any relevant toxicological data available for molybdenum, iron or any other residual elements [7].

It is hard to assess the problem of allergological effects since the epicutan tests do not allow for conclusions to be made automatically as far as the reactions in the joint area are concerned. On the other hand, any surgical tools used in operations will leave behind undesired metal traces (which can be detected either histochemically or as foreign bodies/susceptibility artefacts in nuclear magnetic tomography).

Assessment of the risks posed by surgical implants made of cobalt-based materials:

The linear abrasion rate exhibited by metal on metal prostheses is lower than the one observed for ceramic or metal on polyethylene systems by the power of ten, but is almost twice as high as the one offered by ceramics on ceramics systems. Apart from that, metal abrasion will not cause osteolysis like PE debris, and hence this combination seems to be perfectly suited for use in arthroplasty. However, metal abrasion particles are frequently discussed in connection with the occurrence of allergic reactions and the risk of cancer. In the beginning, high abrasion levels usually will be detected, which even after lapse of the run-in phase cause increased chromium concentrations in the serum and increased chromium and cobalt discharge rates. The things which seem to be more alarming are the results obtained from whole-blood measurements and the detection of metal particles in tissues located far away from the prosthesis. It can be concluded from the published data so far that particles are released from the alloys as a result of fretting corrosion, and that such particles remain stable for reasons of the alloy's position in the electrochemical series. Only a minor fraction will be susceptible to contact corrosion as a result of which it will enter into chemical reactions. The measurements did not yield any significant increase in serum cobalt concentrations. Apart from that, cobalt represents an indispensable element of the human metabolism. Although the chromium levels in the serum were found to have increased, there weren't any toxic levels observed.

Also, the fear that metal implants may cause malignant tumours, which has been expressed time and again, has not been confirmed by long-term studies. The manufacturers of such implants are right in pointing out to their own investigations [4, 14]. An increase in the tumour risk as a result of metal abrasion from metal on metal THRs has not been confirmed neither by the data of the International Agency for Research on Cancer [7] nor by the studies conducted by Visuri et al. which covered a period of 15 years [17]. Also, there aren't any genetic defects to be expected as a result of the measured serum levels [6]. With today's state of knowledge, metal abrasion particles released from resurfacing prostheses made of cobalt-based alloys will not pose any special risk not even in younger patients (also including female patients capable of childbearing). On the other hand, there are excellent clinical results obtained from the implantation of resurfacing prostheses (fig. 5). Conservation of the proximal femur also offers long-term benefits particularly to younger patients since the possibility of revision offered by such prostheses in the case of complications is much better than the one offered by conventional stem-type prostheses. As long as there aren't any better materials available for the purpose of resurfacing, the theoretical risk posed by metal abrasion can be disregarded in view of the clinical benefits offered by resurfacing prostheses since there haven't been any harmful effects of metal abrasion detected so far.

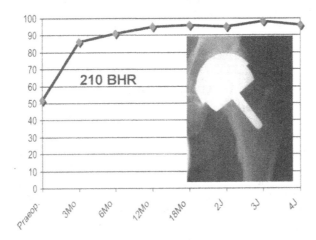

Figure 5:
Curve of the Harris-Hip-Score subsequent to implantation of a metal on metal resurfacing prosthesis.

References

1. Amstutz, HC, P Grigoris (1996) Metal on Metal Bearings in Hip Arthroplasty. Clin Orthop 329S, S11-S34
2. Anonym (o.J.) The Century in Orthopedics.
   www.slackinc.com/bone/ortoday/200001/time.pdf
3. Band T (2003) Microstructure and Metallurgy for Metal on Metal Bearings. The International Resurfacing Forum, June 13th –15th, Malaga
4. Centerpulse (o.J) MetasulR Metal Ion Studies. www.centerpulse.com
5. Elke R (2001) Partikelkrankheit. Orthopäde 30, 258 – 265
6. Expert Group on Vitamins and Minerals (2002) Review of Cobalt/Chromium
   www.foodstandards.gov.uk

7. International Agency for Research on Cancer (1999) IARC Monographs on the Evaluation of Carcinogenic Risks to Humans: Surgical Implants and other Foreign Bodies (Vol. 74) http://monographs.iarc.fr/htdocs/monographs/vol74/implants.html

8. Jacobs JJ, AK Doorn, et al. (1996) Cobalt and Chromium Concentrations in Patients with Metal-on-Metal total Hip Replacements. 5th World Biomaterial Congress, June 2, 1996, Toronto, 918

9. Lhotka C, J Steffan et al. (2000) Determination of Cobalt and Chromium Blood Concentrations in Patients with different Metal-Metal Pairings. AAOS Meeting Orlando, March 17, 2000

10. Jacobsson SA, D Krister, O Wahlström (1996) 20-Year Results of McKee-Farrar Versus Charnley Prosthesis. Cin Orthop 329S, S60-S68

11. Maltoni C, F Minardi,, JF Holland (o.J.) Physical Carcinogens. www.cancer.org

12. McMinn DJW (2003) Die Entwicklung des Metall/Metall-Hüftoberflächenersatzes. Hip International 13 (Suppl. 2)

13. National Institute for Clinical Excellence (2002) Guidance on the use of metal on metal hip resurfacing arthroplasty. Technology Appraisal Guidance No 44. www.nice.org.uk

14. SulzerMedica (1999) Research and Analysis News: Total Joint Replacement and Cancer. Firmenmitteilung

15. Ungethüm, M, W Winkler-Gnieweck (1984) Metallische Werkstoffe in der Orthopädie und Unfallchirurgie. Thieme, Stuttgart

16. Varano R, JD Bobyn, S Yue (2003) Does Alloy Heat Treatment Influence Metal-on-Metal Wear? Orthop Res Soc Poster #1399 49th Annual Meeting

17. Visuri T, et al. (1996) Cancer Risk After Metal on Metal and Polyethylene on Metal Total Hip Arthroplasty. Clin Orthop 329S, S280-9

18. Weber, BG (1992) Metall-Metall-Totalprothese des Hüftgelenkes: Zurück in die Zukunft. Z Orthop 130, 306-309

3.9 Surface Replacement of the Hip: Contra

S. Goebel, M. Blanke and Ch. Hendrich

Introduction

The surface replacement of the hip as an alternative method to the implantation of a conventional hip prosthesis seems to be advantageous in consideration to bone conservation particularly for young patients.

Because of the today's commonly used materials and designs there is almost no aseptic loosening of the acetabular side to be seen. Therefore the conservation of the bone stock of the femur might be the major profit of a surface replacement.

Earlier variations of the surface replacement prosthesis such as the Wagner cap used polyethylene components for the acetabular cup. In fact of the large head diameter only thin polyethylene components could be used. This is said to be the major cause for the failure of the Wagner cap. In consideration of this fact the use of hard material for the articulation is necessary. Today there is a large amount of just metal to metal surface replacement designs on the market, however there are no alternative materials available yet.

Aseptic loosening

Clinical datas of the surface replacement of the hip published in the literature are leaving open many questions. For the Wagner prosthesis a 12.4 % loosening rate in 466 with a follow-up period of 7 years has been described.[16] Dustmann et al. showed a loosening rate of 9 % after 3 years.[14] Solely Wagner himself described only 6 loosenings of components during a follow-up of 4 months to 4 years.[57]

Beside the aseptic loosening of the surface replacement of the hip because of the thin polyethylene component there was a second reason identified. A necrosis of the femoral head underneath the cap is considered to be another major cause of implant loosening.[24]

The BHR-prosthesis by McMinn for the different designs showed loosing rates of 7 % within a follow-up period of 2.8 years for the cemented version and up to 8.6 % within a follow-up period of 4.2 years for the press-fit group.[39]

For the THARIES prosthesis, a metal-polyethylene surface replacement design, Amstutz et al. reported a 10 years survivorship ratio of merely 48 %. In 97 % of the cases an aseptic loosening of either one or even both components was found. Because of this metal-on-metal components were used. For this design 4 year survivorship rates of 94.4 % are reported. 10 of 12 revisions were due to either aseptic loosening of the femoral component or to fracture of the femoral neck.[2]

In contrast in today's models problems with the acetabular shell are almost none existing. The high rates of aseptic loosening are almost exclusively based on failures of the femoral component.

In sight of the cited literature there are still studies missing with sufficient number of patients and follow-up time.

In comparison the new generation of the ceramic-on-ceramic components show good results. In a recent a 97.5 % survivorship rate for a young and active group (average age was 41 years) during a follow-up period of 5 years was traced. The 10 year follow-up showed a rate of 89.4 % for 131 total hip endoprostheses.[50] In another study there were 85 % of uncemented ceramic-on-ceramic total hip prostheses implanted during the years 1979 and 1980 without any aseptic loosening after 18.5 years of follow up.[22] Lazzaro et al. showed a survivor-ship rate of 81.2 % after 13 years. They reviewed 38 patients with an average age of 55 years.[33] In a recent publication, no aseptic loosening occurred after 5 to 8 years of follow-up.[26]

Nizard described that in the first years of usage of the ceramic-on-ceramic components there were a few cases of broken ceramic components seen. However, with improved materials no further cases of this specific complication were reported.[42]

Wear behavior

The wear of the polyethylene is the main reason for osteolysis around the prosthesis resulting in the aseptic loosening.[19,25,41] The wear rate increases with larger head sizes.[12,30,31,36,46] For surface replacement hip prosthesis large head sizes are used. First attempts with a metal-polyethylene combination by the THARIES-prosthesis had to be stopped.[5] Metal-on-metal-components can supposed to generate less wear compared to metal-polyethylene- or ceramic-polyethylene-components.[5] However, a metal-on-metal wear couple results in a higher concentration of cobalt and chrome in the serum and urine.[28,29,47] Relative to a possible carcinogenesis of cobalt-chrome-molybdenum particles a study by Memoli et al. suggests a slight increase in the rate of sarcomas.[40] Visuri et al. found a 1.23 times higher incidence for carcinomas by patients supplied with metal-on-metal-prostheses.[56] Furthermore there was a significant increase for kidney- and prostate-carcinomas and also for lymphomas and leukemias. [18,44] Other studies could not underline these findings.[17,23,35,45,54] Other unwanted side-effects, for example the decrease in white blood cells[48], sensibilisation of lymphocytes and the increase of inflammatory cytokines were described.[20] To summarize, long term studies have to be performed to verify the unwished effects of the metal wear and the increase of the concentration the ion-concentration in the blood and urine. Clinical data for the metal-on-metal prosthesis with large head diameter are missing, yet.

In contrast the ceramic-on-ceramic wear couple regarded as bioinert. Toxic effects have not been described yet during 40 years of use.[9,13,60]

Revision of surface replacement prosthesis

The advantage of a surface replacement prosthesis may be a better conservation of bone stock, especially in regard to the head and the neck of the femur.[4,5,58]

This conserved bone stock should result in an easier revision procedure. In today's literature there are just three papers dealing with the outcome of revision of surface replacement prosthesis of the hip. Steele et al. performed 13 revision surgeries in 12 patients after a surface replacement. The average follow-up was 3 years after the revision. The results showed a comparable outcome between the revisions after surface replacement and the revision after a conventional hip arthoplasty.[53] Thomas and Amstutz analyzed 17 revisions, of which 8 patients were supplied with a conventional and 9 patients with a surface replacement hip prostheses. They found no significant improvement of the clinical outcome when comparing both groups. On the one hand they described an easier revision on the femoral side. Conversely the difficulties with acetabular component revision seemed to be higher as for a revision of the conventional prosthesis.[55] In particular the rough coated press-fit acetabular shell of the metal-on-metal surface replacement made revisions more difficult. Capello et al. found in 24 patients after revision of a surface replacement prosthesis a lower rate of complications in comparison to revisions after conventional hip arthroplasty.[7] Ultimately only one study showing an advantage for the revision of the surface replacement.

Modern concepts with metal-on-metal wear couples are using large head sizes. Nevertheless there is always a bedding-in period of the head and cup. The effect of a second bedding-in period after a revision using a larger revision head has not been investigates either in simulator studies nor in vivo.

Dislocation and leg length

The advantage of large heads in the hip arthroplasty is evident in a higher range-of-motion, the avoidance of impingement and lower rates of dislocation.[8,11,15,32]

For the surface replacement the cited literature has fulfilled the expectations relative to the dislocation rate. Amstutz describes a dislocation rate of 0.75 % in 400 patients. The range of motion could also be improved significantly.[1]

Similar results, however, can also be performed with a modern ceramic-on-ceramic hip prosthesis. In an own study with 40 patients only one dislocation occurred. However the postoperative range-of-motion was inferior compared to the study of Amstutz.

However, today there are ceramic-on-ceramic prostheses available with a head size of 36 mm in combination with a 12/14 mm cone which allows an increase of the range-of-motion of more than 10 %. The head-neck-ratio is considered to play the major role for the quantity of the range-of-motion.[10,37]

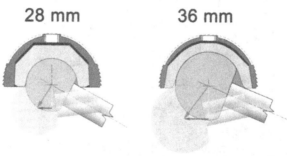

28 mm   **36 mm**

Figure 1:
36 mm large ceramic-on-ceramic wear couples to obtain more stable THA with a higher range-of-motion with permission from Toni, A., G. Willman; Bioceramics in Joint Arthroplasty; Georg Thieme Verlag; New York Stuttgart 2001.

Amstutz et al. describe the leg length difference after implantation of surface replacement hip prosthesis. There was a difference of 1-2 cm in 4 % of the patients, 2 % had a difference of 2-3 cm and even one patient showed a difference of more than 3 cm. The rather poor results might depend on the more difficult intraoperative testing by using the posterior approach.[3] In our own study all patients except one showed a leg length difference within 1 cm by using the transgluteal approach.

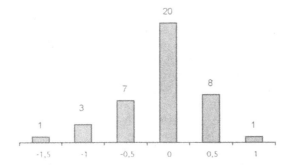

Figure 2:
Leg-length difference postoperatively in cm of 40 patients with a ceramic-on-ceramic arthroplasty.
The only patient with a leg-length inequability of 1.5 cm had a shortening of –3.5 cm pre-operatively.

Surgical approach

For the implantation of a surface replacement large surgical approaches are needed to create a good overview of the acetabular region. Wagner described an anterior approach[59] whereas Amstutz and McMinn prefer the posterior approach.[5,38] For this approach the proximal femur is mobilized ventrally. Paresis of the femoralis nerve occur in 1 % of the cases, Amstutz. (personal communication)

In today's hip arthoplasty minimal-invasive approaches become more and more interesting because of their preservation of the soft tissue, faster rehabilitation and better cosmetics.[52,61] In conventional hip arthoplasty a surgical approach of 7 – 12 cm or a two-incision technique may be performed. Because of the above mentioned reasons for surface replacement a large posterior approach is necessary.

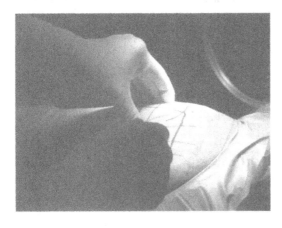

Figure 3:
Large posterior approach.

This stands in a certain opposition to the minimal-invasive rationale of this technique.

Restrictive to a final estimation is the fact that there are not many studies about the minimal-invasive approaches available so far. However because of the lack of sufficient studies employing minimal-invasive techniques a decisive statement about its usefulness cannot be made, yet.

Conclusion

With a 5-year survivorship-rate of up to 95 % even among the modern surface replacement prosthesis the loosening rate is worse than for the conventional total hip arthoplasty even in a young patient group. IN contrast, for the ceramic-on-ceramic prostheses 5-years survivor ship-rates of 97.5 % to 100 % and 10-year rates of 82 % to 89 % have been published.[6,21,27,34,43,49,51]

Modern surface replacement prostheses are available as metal-on-metal combinations only. For longer bearings no clinical results for the wear rate are available, yet. Additionally, one has to consider the increasing concentration of metal-ions in the serum and urine. The long term side-effect are not know, yet. In contrast the ceramic materials have not shown any biological side-effects during 40 years of usage.

The surface replacement of the hip promises a better bone stock for a future revision. An advantage on outcome has only been shown in one of three studies. For the range of motion the modern surface replacement has proved a better result. On the other hand 36 mm ceramic heads in combination with a 12/14 mm cone are available allowing a similar range-of-motion. Especially with regard to the leg-length difference the ceramic-on-ceramic prosthesis shows a superior result compared to a surface replacement.

For the implantation of a surface replacement large posterior approach is necessary. This is in direct contrast to its minimal-invasive goal. In contrast ceramic-on-ceramic prostheses can favorably implanted using minimal-invasive techniques.

References

1. Amstutz HC, Beaule PE, Dorey FJ, Le Duff MJ, Campbell PA, Gruen TA: Metal-on-Metal Hybrid Surface Arthroplasty: Two to Six-Year Follow-up Study. J Bone Joint Surg Am 86-A:28-39, 2004
2. Amstutz HC, Beaule PE, Dorey FJ, Le Duff MJ, Campbell PA, Gruen TA: Metal-on-Metal Hybrid Surface Arthroplasty: Two to Six-Year Follow-up Study. J Bone Joint Surg Am 86-A:28-39, 2004
3. Amstutz HC, Beaule PE, Dorey FJ, Le Duff MJ, Campbell PA, Gruen TA: Metal-on-Metal Hybrid Surface Arthroplasty: Two to Six-Year Follow-up Study. J Bone Joint Surg Am 86-A:28-39, 2004
4. Amstutz HC, Dorey F, O'Carroll PF: THARIES resurfacing arthroplasty. Evolution and long-term results. Clin Orthop92-114, 1986
5. Amstutz HC, Grigoris P, Dorey FJ: Evolution and future of surface replacement of the hip. J Orthop Sci 3:169-186, 1998
6. Boehler M, Knahr K, Plenk H, Jr., Walter A, Salzer M, Schreiber V: Long-term results of uncemented alumina acetabular implants. J Bone Joint Surg Br 76:53-59, 1994

7. Capello WN, Trancik TM, Misamore G, Eaton R: Analysis of revision surgery of resurfacing hip arthroplasty. Clin Orthop50-55, 1982

8. Chandler DR, Glousman R, Hull D, McGuire PJ, Kim IS, Clarke IC, Sarmiento A: Prosthetic hip range of motion and impingement. The effects of head and neck geometry. Clin Orthop284-291, 1982

9. Christel PS: Biocompatibility of surgical-grade dense polycrystalline alumina. Clin Orthop10-18, 1992

10. D'Lima DD, Urquhart AG, Buehler KO, Walker RH, Colwell CW, Jr.: The effect of the orientation of the acetabular and femoral components on the range of motion of the hip at different head-neck ratios. J Bone Joint Surg Am 82:315-321, 2000

11. D'Lima DD, Urquhart AG, Buehler KO, Walker RH, Colwell CW, Jr.: The effect of the orientation of the acetabular and femoral components on the range of motion of the hip at different head-neck ratios. J Bone Joint Surg Am 82:315-321, 2000

12. Devane PA, Horne JG: Assessment of polyethylene wear in total hip replacement. Clin Orthop59-72, 1999

13. Dorlot JM: Long-term effects of alumina components in total hip prostheses. Clin Orthop47-52, 1992

14. Dustmann HO, Godolias G: [Experiences with Wagner's hip joint cup endoprosthesis. Indication, results complications]. Z Orthop Ihre Grenzgeb 122:106-113, 1984

15. Elfick AP, Hall RM, Pinder IM, Unsworth A: Wear in retrieved acetabular components: effect of femoral head radius and patient parameters. J Arthroplasty 13:291-295, 1998

16. Ferdini R, Moos N, Brunner H: [Experience with 466 re-examined Wagner double-cup hip joint endoprostheses]. Z Orthop Ihre Grenzgeb 124:740-742, 1986

17. Gaechter A, Alroy J, Andersson GB, Galante J, Rostoker W, Schajowicz F: Metal carcinogenesis: a study of the carcinogenic activity of solid metal alloys in rats. J Bone Joint Surg Am 59:622-624, 1977

18. Gillespie WJ, Henry DA, O'Connell DL, Kendrick S, Juszczak E, McInneny K, Derby L: Development of hematopoietic cancers after implantation of total joint replacement. Clin OrthopS290-S296, 1996

19. Goldberg VM, Ninomiya J, Kelly G, Kraay M: Hybrid total hip arthroplasty: a 7- to 11-year followup. Clin Orthop147-154, 1996

20. Granchi D, Ciapetti G, Savarino L, Stea S, Filippini F, Sudanese A, Rotini R, Giunti A: Expression of the CD69 activation antigen on lymphocytes of patients with hip prosthesis. Biomaterials 21:2059-2065, 2000

21. Hamadouche M, Boutin P, Daussange J, Bolander ME, Sedel L: Alumina-on-alumina total hip arthroplasty: a minimum 18.5-year follow-up study. J Bone Joint Surg Am 84-A:69-77, 2002

22. Hamadouche M, Boutin P, Daussange J, Bolander ME, Sedel L: Alumina-on-alumina total hip arthroplasty: a minimum 18.5-year follow-up study. J Bone Joint Surg Am 84-A:69-77, 2002

23. Howie DW, Rogers SD, McGee MA, Haynes DR: Biologic effects of cobalt chrome in cell and animal models. Clin OrthopS217-S232, 1996

24. Huiskes R, Strens PH, van Heck J, Slooff TJ: Interface stresses in the resurfaced hip. Finite element analysis of load transmission in the femoral head. Acta Orthop Scand 56:474-478, 1985

25. Huk OL, Bansal M, Betts F, Rimnac CM, Lieberman JR, Huo MH, Salvati EA: Polyethylene and metal debris generated by non-articulating surfaces of modular acetabular components. J Bone Joint Surg Br 76:568-574, 1994

26. Huo MH, Martin RP, Zatorski LE, Keggi KJ: Cementless total hip arthroplasties using ceramic-on-ceramic articulation in young patients. A minimum 5-year follow-up study. J Arthroplasty 11:673-678, 1996

27. Hyder N, Nevelos AB, Barabas TG: Cementless ceramic hip arthroplasties in patients less than 30 years old. J Arthroplasty 11:679-686, 1996

28. Jacobs JJ, Skipor AK, Doorn PF, Campbell P, Schmalzried TP, Black J, Amstutz HC: Cobalt and chromium concentrations in patients with metal on metal total hip replacements. Clin OrthopS256-S263, 1996

29. Jacobs JJ, Skipor AK, Patterson LM, Hallab NJ, Paprosky WG, Black J, Galante JO: Metal release in patients who have had a primary total hip arthroplasty. A prospective, controlled, longitudinal study. J Bone Joint Surg Am 80:1447-1458, 1998

30. Jasty M, Goetz DD, Bragdon CR, Lee KR, Hanson AE, Elder JR, Harris WH: Wear of polyethylene acetabular components in total hip arthroplasty. An analysis of one hundred and twenty-eight components retrieved at autopsy or revision operations. J Bone Joint Surg Am 79:349-358, 1997

31. Kawamura H, Bourne RB, Dunbar MJ, Rorabeck CH: Polyethylene wear of the porous-coated anatomic total hip arthroplasty with an average 11-year follow-up. J Arthroplasty 16:116-121, 2001

32. Krushell RJ, Burke DW, Harris WH: Range of motion in contemporary total hip arthroplasty. The impact of modular head-neck components. J Arthroplasty 6:97-101, 1991

33. Lazzaro F, Verdoia C, Gorla P, Balbino C, Benvenuti R: Ceramic-ceramic in total hip arthroplasty. An analysis of 7-13 year survival rate. Chir Organi Mov 84:319-328, 1999

34. Lazzaro F, Verdoia C, Gorla P, Balbino C, Benvenuti R: Ceramic-ceramic in total hip arthroplasty. An analysis of 7-13 year survival rate. Chir Organi Mov 84:319-328, 1999

35. Lewis CG, Belniak RM, Hopfer SM, Sunderman FW, Jr.: Cobalt in periprosthetic soft tissue. Observations in 6 revision cases. Acta Orthop Scand 62:447-450, 1991

36. Livermore J, Ilstrup D, Morrey B: Effect of femoral head size on wear of the polyethylene acetabular component. J Bone Joint Surg Am 72:518-528, 1990

37. Mahoney CR, Pellicci PM: Complications in primary total hip arthroplasty: avoidance and management of dislocations. Instr Course Lect 52:247-255, 2003

38. McMinn D, Treacy R, Lin K, Pynsent P: Metal on metal surface replacement of the hip. Experience of the McMinn prothesis. Clin OrthopS89-S98, 1996

39. McMinn D, Treacy R, Lin K, Pynsent P: Metal on metal surface replacement of the hip. Experience of the McMinn prothesis. Clin OrthopS89-S98, 1996

40. Memoli VA, Urban RM, Alroy J, Galante JO: Malignant neoplasms associated with orthopedic implant materials in rats. J Orthop Res 4:346-355, 1986

41. Murray DW, Rushton N: Macrophages stimulate bone resorption when they phagocytose particles. J Bone Joint Surg Br 72:988-992, 1990

42. Nizard RS, Sedel L, Christel P, Meunier A, Soudry M, Witvoet J: Ten-year survivorship of cemented ceramic-ceramic total hip prosthesis. Clin Orthop53-63, 1992

43. Nizard RS, Sedel L, Christel P, Meunier A, Soudry M, Witvoet J: Ten-year survivorship of cemented ceramic-ceramic total hip prosthesis. Clin Orthop53-63, 1992

44. Nyren O, McLaughlin JK, Gridley G, Ekbom A, Johnell O, Fraumeni JF, Jr., Adami HO: Cancer risk after hip replacement with metal implants: a population-based cohort study in Sweden. J Natl Cancer Inst 87:28-33, 1995

45. Paavolainen P, Pukkala E, Pulkkinen P, Visuri T: Cancer incidence in Finnish hip replacement patients from 1980 to 1995: a nationwide cohort study involving 31,651 patients. J Arthroplasty 14:272-280, 1999

46. Pedersen DR, Callaghan JJ, Johnston TL, Fetzer GB, Johnston RC: Comparison of femoral head penetration rates between cementless acetabular components with 22-mm and 28-mm heads. J Arthroplasty 16:111-115, 2001

47. Savarino L, Granchi D, Ciapetti G, Cenni E, Greco M, Rotini R, Veronesi CA, Baldini N, Giunti A: Ion release in stable hip arthroplasties using metal-on-metal articulating surfaces: a comparison between short- and medium-term results. J Biomed Mater Res 66A:450-456, 2003

48. Savarino L, Granchi D, Ciapetti G, Cenni E, Greco M, Rotini R, Veronesi CA, Baldini N, Giunti A: Ion release in stable hip arthroplasties using metal-on-metal articulating surfaces: a comparison between short- and medium-term results. J Biomed Mater Res 66A:450-456, 2003

49. Sedel L, Kerboull L, Christel P, Meunier A, Witvoet J: Alumina-on-alumina hip replacement. Results and survivorship in young patients. J Bone Joint Surg Br 72:658-663, 1990

50. Sedel L, Nizard RS, Kerboull L, Witvoet J: Alumina-alumina hip replacement in patients younger than 50 years old. Clin Orthop175-183, 1994

51. Sedel L, Nizard RS, Kerboull L, Witvoet J: Alumina-alumina hip replacement in patients younger than 50 years old. Clin Orthop175-183, 1994

52. Sherry E, Egan M, Warnke PH, Henderson A, Eslick GD: Minimal invasive surgery for hip

53. Steele RA, Dempster D, Smith MA: Total hip replacement of failed surface arthroplasty. Acta Orthop Scand 56:133-134, 1985

54. Tharani R, Dorey FJ, Schmalzried TP: The risk of cancer following total hip or knee arthroplasty. J Bone Joint Surg Am 83-A:774-780, 2001

55. Thomas BJ, Amstutz HC: Revision surgery for failed surface arthroplasty of the hip. Clin Orthop42-49, 1982

56. Visuri T, Pukkala E, Paavolainen P, Pulkkinen P, Riska EB: Cancer risk after metal on metal and polyethylene on metal total hip arthroplasty. Clin OrthopS280-S289, 1996

57. Wagner H: Surface replacement arthroplasty of the hip. Clin Orthop102-130, 1978

58. Walter A: On the material and the tribology of alumina-alumina couplings for hip joint prostheses. Clin Orthop31-46, 1992

59. Wenz JF, Gurkan I, Jibodh SR: Mini-incision total hip arthroplasty: a comparative assessment of perioperative outcomes. Orthopedics 25:1031-1043, 2002

Hip Revisions with Ceramic Solutions

4.1 The Concept of CeramTec to Offer Ball Heads Dedicated to Hip Revision Demands

P. Merkert

Aim

Ceramic ball heads are used since 30 years in hip endoprostheses. In the case of a revision where the ball head needs to be exchanged but the stem is fixed, only limited solutions are available on the market. Up to date CeramTec advised not to implant a ceramic ball head on a used stem.

CeramTec has decided to provide a revision solution for this case. This shall give the surgeon the possibility to use a ceramic ball head in a revision case where the stem is fixed in the femur for either a ceramic wear couple solution or a system with a PE insert.

Concept of a Ceramic Revision Ball Head

In revisions where the stem is not exchanged there is always the possibility that the stem is damaged for example by removing the ball head from the stem. A potential damage of the stem will induce a stress concentration when a ceramic ball head is placed directly on the damaged taper which could lead to a breakage of the ceramic ball. Therefore CeramTec has decided to use a system with a metal sleeve (figure 1).

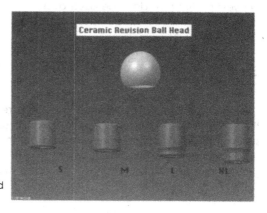

Figure 1:
Concept of ceramic revision ball head with metal sleeve.

The sleeve will be adapted on the taper of the stem which creates a new taper size where the ceramic ball head is put on. The first solution CeramTec wants to place on the market is for 12/14 tapers. Possible neck lengths are S, M, L and also XL which will be realized through different metal sleeves. It is planned to have first two ceramic ball head sizes: 28 mm and 32 mm with one standard taper. Further tapers and other outer diameters (36 mm) will be evaluated.

Ceramic Revision Ball Head with Stem

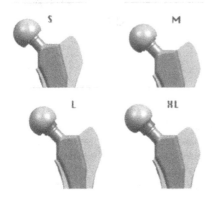

Figure 2:
Combination of ceramic revision ball head with stem.

Development and Test Concept for the Ceramic Revision Ball Head at CeramTec

The development of a ceramic revision ball head at CeramTec is devided in two major stages. The first stage is dedicated to understand the system of all three components, find limitations to the system and to define the manufacturing standard for the revision ball head. In this phase a large amount of evaluation and validation in production as well as testing in different settings are the major parts. At the end of this stage it should be clear how the ceramic revision ball head is produced and that all necessary processes are validated. The testing involves questions like what is the influence of the metal sleeve or a damage at the taper for the mechanical properties, what are the worst case settings and so on. The answers should provide a detailed overview of the system and how customer projects can be conducted. The second stage will deal with defined customer projects.

Conclusion

During 2004 CeramTec will offer a ceramic revision ball heads system to give the surgeon the opportunity to use ceramic solutions in revisions. The revision system consists of a metal sleeve and a ceramic ball head. The release of the product undergoes two development stages: the first stage to find answers to general question and a second stage where customer projects will be handled.

4.2 Clinical and Technical Aspects in THA-Revision Surgery: Current Problems, Guidelines for Current and Future Solutions

H. Kienapfel

Introduction

In total hip revision arthroplasty each case offers the surgeon the possibility to use an implant system in combination with an operative technique matching the new standards of implant technology and evidence based medicine. The objective of this presentation is to demonstrate a consensus-based revision strategy for all possible revision scenarios.

Materials and Methods

All possible revision scenarios were subdivided in 12 different revision-causes which were linked to either the acetabular or the stem component. Subsequently 12 guide-line tables were developed. Each table demonstrates for each revision scenario the typical current revision procedure and the potential advantages using a new ceramic revision ball system.

Results

The reasons for the current procedures and the new ceramic ball system are systematically reviewed and discussed. As an example Table 1 demonstrates the current and future revision strategy in the case of aseptic loosening and/or mechanical failure of the acetabular component.

Figures 1, 2 ond 3 demonstrate an example of acetabular bar leading to mechanical failure.

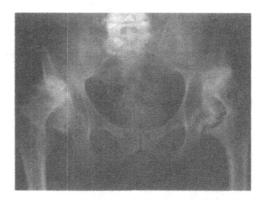

Figure 1:
Preoperative radiographs of secondary OA due to hip dysplasia (DDH).

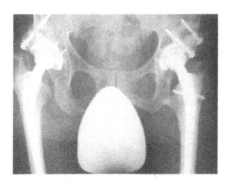 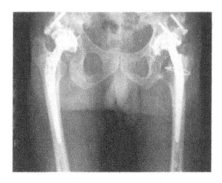

Figure 2:
Postoperative radiographs after hybrid THA
with femoral head autograft acetabular roof
augmentation.

Figure 3:
Mechanical failure of the left acetabular
component.

Table 1:
Recommendations in case of aseptic loosening of the acetabular component.

Revision cause	Stem / Cup	Typical current procedure	Why?	Procedure with ceramic revision head	Why?
Aseptic	Stem can remain in situ	1. Removal of head component	♣)	1. Removal of head component.	♠)
Loosening		2. New acetabular component or new PE-Liner		2. New acetabular component or new PE-Liner	
Acetabular Component		3. Ceramic head should not be used. Metal-head is preferrably used if inspection and palpation of the stem taper does not demonstrate any damage.		3. Ceramic revision head is recommended.	°)

♣) During the disengagement of the head component – both with metal and ceramic heads – the surface structure of the stem taper will be damaged. If a ceramic head would be used, there is an increased risk of breakage. Within the conically shaped ceramic ball hoop stress concentrations can develop based on the surface damage of the stem taper.

♠) If the articulation partners Ceramic / PE or Ceramic/Ceramic are used a decreased wear rate can be expected eventually leading to a reduced revision rate and to a longer implant survival.

°) If the articulation partners Ceramic/Ceramic are used the three body wear problem will be excluded.

If in addition considerable damage of the stem taper can be seen either metal heads were used or the stem was exchanged. Now the revision ceramic ball system offers a new solution (fig. 4, 5).

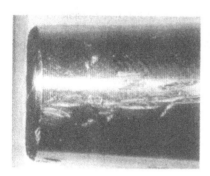

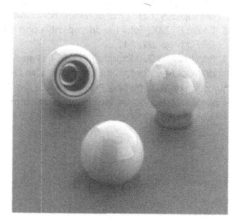

Figure 4:
Damage of the stem taper.

Figure 5:
Revision Ceramic ball system can be used as a new solution to provide a reduced future wear burden.

Discussion

Advantages and disadvantages of different revision strategies will be discussed in detail for all revision causes represented in 12 guideline tables and for each revision table literature references will be given.

Conclusion

To reduce the wear problem the articulation partners of ceramic and poyethylene or ceramic in combination with ceramic are an excellent choice. The new ceramic ball system offers substantial advantages when compared to current revision strategies.

References

1. Amis AA (1996) Is polyethylene still the best prosthetic bearing surface? J Bone Joint Surg Br 78: 345-348
2. Archibeck MJ, Jacobs JJ, Black J (2000) Alternate bearing surfaces in total joint arthroplasty: biological considerations. Clin Orthop 379: 12-21
3. Boutin P (2000) Total hip arthroplasty using a ceramic prosthesis. Pierre Boutin (1924-1989). Clin Orthop 379: 3-11
4. Paprosky WG, Magnus RE (1994) Principles of bone grafting in revision total hip arthroplasty. Acetabular technique. Clin Orthop 298: 147-155
5. Paprosky WG, Perona PG, Lawrence JM (1994) Acetabular defect classification and surgical reconstruction in revision arthroplasty. A 6-year follow-up evaluation. J Arthroplasty 9: 33-44

SESSION 5

**THR Instability and Dislocation:
Different Solutions in THR**

5.1 Risk Factors for Dislocation after Total Hip Arthroplasty: Results of a Long Term Analysis

D. J. Berry

Part I: The Cumulative Long-Term Risk of Dislocation after Primary Charnley Total Hip Arthroplasty

Introduction

A wide variable prevalence of dislocation after total hip arthroplasty (THA) has been reported, partly because of the variable lengths of follow-up for this specific endpoint. The effect of patient demographic factors on long-term risk of dislocation as a function of time after THA has not been well understood. The purpose of this study was to determine the risk of dislocation following cemented Charnley total hip arthroplasty with a 22 mm head size as a function of time and to investigate the patient demographic factors that influence the cumulative dislocation risk and time dependency of dislocation risk.

Materials and Methods

6621 consecutive primary Charnley THA performed in 2868 women and 2589 men (mean age 63 years, range 13-95 years) were performed at one institution between 1969 and 1984. Patients were followed at routine intervals and specifically queried about dislocation. The cumulative risk of dislocation was calculated using the Kaplan-Meier method.

Results

320 of the hips (4.8%) dislocated. The cumulative risk of a first time dislocation was 1% at one month, 1.9% at one year and then rose at a constant rate of approximately 1% every five years (0.2% per year) to 7% at 25 years for patients that were alive and unrevised at that time. In a multivariate analysis, the relative risk of dislocation for female (versus male) patients was 2.1, and for patients greater than or equal to 70 (compared to those less than 70) was 1.3. Three underlying diagnosis groups had a significantly higher risk of dislocation than osteoarthritis: osteonecrosis of the femoral head, acute or nonunited fracture of the proximal femur, and inflammatory arthritis.

Conclusions

The cumulative long-term risk of dislocation after THA is considerably greater than reported in short-term studies. The incidence of dislocation is highest in the first year after arthroplasty then continues at a relatively constant level for the life of the arthroplasty. Patients at highest risk are women and patients with a diagnosis of osteonecrosis of the femoral head or acute or nonunited proximal femur fracture.

Reference
Berry DJ; von Knoch M; Schleck CD; Harmsen WS: The Cumulative Long-Term Risk of Dislocation after Primary Charnley Total Hip Arthroplasty. J Bone Joint Surg Am, January 2004.

Part II: The Long-Term Cumulative Risk of Dislocation After Primary Total Hip Arthroplasty: Effect of Femoral Head Size and Operative Approach

Purpose

To determine the effect of femoral head size and operative approach on long-term cumulative risk of dislocation after primary THA.

Materials and Methods

From 1969-1999, 22,174 primary THAs were performed at a single institution. Patients routinely were followed at defined intervals and specifically queried about dislocation. Operative approach was anterolateral in 10,186, posterolateral in 3710, and transtrochanteric in 8278. Femoral head size was 22 mm in 8641, 26 mm in 1123, 28 mm in 8791, and 32 mm in 3515.

Results

918 of 22,174 hips (4.1%) had at least one dislocation. The cumulative risk of dislocation for the whole group was 2.2% at one year, 3% at five years, and 6% at 20 years. The cumulative 15-year risk of dislocation was 4.2% for anterolateral, 7.9% for posterolateral (Hazard ratio 2.2), and 4.5% for transtrochanteric approach (Hazard ratio 1.1)(p<0.001). The ten-year cumulative probability of at least one dislocation for the anterior approach was 3.9% for the 22 mm heads, 3.0% for 28 mm heads, and 2.4% for 32 mm heads, and for the posterior approach was 12.2% for the 22 mm heads, 6.9% for 28 mm heads, and 3.5% for 32 mm heads.

In the multivariate model the hazard ratio for dislocation for 22 mm heads compared to 32 mm heads was 1.7 (95% confidence interval, 1.4 to 2.2: p<0.0001); for 28 mm heads compared to 32 mm heads was 1.3 (95% confidence interval, 1.0 to 1.6; p=0.025).

Conclusions

This paper demonstrates that for the 22, 28, and 32 mm femoral heads, larger head size was associated with a lower risk of first time hip dislocation. The posterior approach has a higher dislocation risk than anterolateral or transtrochanteric approach.

Reference
Berry DJ; von Knoch M; Harmsen WS: Presented at the American Academy of Orthopaedic Surgeons annual meeting, 2003.

5.2 Hip-Spine Relationships: A New Concept to Analyse THP Dysfunction and Instability

J.-Y. Lazennec and G. Saillant

Introduction

Dislocation is one of the most common complications of total hip replacement [25, 26]. The period of greatest risk for dislocation has been reported to be within the first few months after surgery, but, even if a hip is stable initially, a first dislocation still can occurs years after surgery.

The concept of cumulative risk factors is widely developed in the literature (type of T.H.P., operative approach, malposition, neurologic impairment, cognitive dysfunction) [2,7,16,18].

For late dislocation, the analysis is often very difficult, and several new mechanical problems are pointed out (muscular deconditioning with time, proximal or rotational migration of the socket and subsidence of the femoral stem reducing soft-tissue tension and increasing osseous impingement) [24].

Repetitive subluxation can be associated with dislocation (early or late) in some patients: subluxation leads to cold flow of the polyethylene of the socket rim and less containment of the femoral head.

In case of early or late dislocation, implant malposition has been reported This risk has been widely documented, using measures of femoral or acetabular anteversion [1,11,21]. But the analysis remains very elementary and especially focused on A.P. views of the pelvis (measuring acetabular frontal inclination) or conventional CT scan datas in patients in supine position.

Lumbosacral pelvic orientation is of outmost importance, as it plays a critical role in the sagittal orientation of the spine and of the hip joints. The trunk equilibrium influences the tridimensionnal orientation of each acetabulum and the functional range of motion of the hips.

The "sagittal spine profile" has been mainly studied by spine surgeons [8,9,11, 12,13].

They observed the side effects of long fusions for scoliosis treatement, without correct adjustment of sagittal plane, leading to more kyphosis and severe disequilibrium.

For a long time, the analysis was mainly focused on lumbar lordosis. The recent studies are more sophisticated, measuring new parameters: they demonstrate that this sagittal equilibrium is the consequence of a postural strategy, specific to each subject.

Duval-Beaupere's studies provided a new dimension to those radiological observations [3]. Each patient is characterized by a "morphological" parameter: the incidence angle (pelvic incidence is the angle between the perpendicular to the sacral plate at its midpoint and the line connecting this point to the midpoint of a line connecting the femoral heads: it represents the thickness of the pelvis). The adaptation of other factors, as "pelvic version" (pelvic tilt) and spinal parameters (sacral tilt, lumbar lordosis, thoracic kyphosis) provides the general conditions for the best adapted posture of the spino-pelvic complex (minimal muscles activity for this "economical" postural situation).

Other studies demonstrated relationship between pelvic and spinal parameters (with a strong correlation between pelvic incidence and sacral slope, pelvic tilt, and lumbar lordosis in a normal population)[5,10,15 ,17,20,23].

Hip-spine relationships

The understanding of this functional anatomy is necessary to explain the strange consequences of some lumbosacral arthrodesis on hip joints and to avoid some difficult adjustments of T.H.P. in patients with a fused or stiff spine.

In the normal subject standing, sitting or lying positions are "instantaneous" situations in a more complex adjustment including spinal movements, sacral tilt and hips flexion [6,19,22]. We often analyse the adaptation for sitting as hip flexion alone, but the lumbosacral movements may create until 30% of the global adjustment. On the contrary, trunk extension is achieved through simultaneous but nonlinear contributions from both the pelvis and lumbar spine throughout the range of motion. (The lumbar spine accounts for 70% of the total, with increased pelvic contributions in initial flexed postures).

Lumbar-pelvic rythm depends on whether the trunk was flexing or extending. During trunk flexion (down lift) there is a greater tendency for lumbar and pelvic rotations to occur simultaneously; during extension (up life) they normally occur more sequentially.

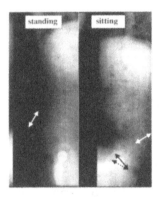

Figure 1:
Lateral views standing and sitting
Modifications of sagittal orientation of the acetabular cups can be observed as well as variation for sacral sagittal tilt.
• In standing position , sacral tilt (ST) is important.
• In sitting position, sacral tilt is low.

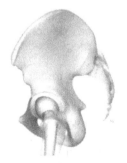 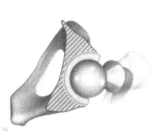

Figure 2:
Standing position.

• On the lateral view, the pelvis is anteverted (forward tilt of the pelvis); the sacrum is relatively horizontal with approximatively 40° sacral tilt (ST).
• On the CT scan, functional acetabular anteversion is low.

Standing position is linked to pelvic anteversion which means anterior tilt of the whole pelvis including the sacrum.

In this situation, the superior endplate of the sacrum on a lateral view creates with the horizontal line the sacral tilt angle ST (mean value 40°).

The acetabulum is oriented in a specific position: we call it "functional anteversion". This "functional anteversion" is the consequence of the "anterior opening" of the acetabulum in the standing position. The "functional anteversion" is not the "morphological anteversion" or "anatomical anteversion" (angle between the margin of the acetabulum and the sagittal plane): this value is a fixed parameter, specific to each subject.

In the standing position, the "functional acetabular anteversion is low" in normal subjects, despite some variations due to different postural patterns.

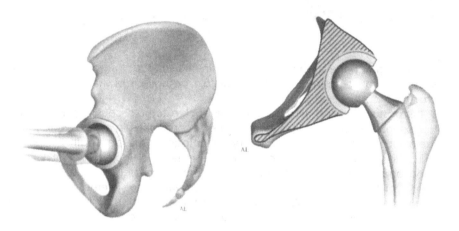

Figure 3:
Sitting position.
- On the lateral view, the pelvis is more retroverted (backward pelvic tilt); the sacrum is more vertical with a low sacral tilting angle (ST).
- On the CT scan, the functional acetabular anteversion is more important.

In sitting position, the situation is the opposite. The pelvis tilts posteriorly according to the progression to the sitting position. The sacral tilt angle (ST) decreases. In a series of more than 350 subjects studied in La Pitié, the ST values were either slightly positive (5° - 10°) or negative.

Sitting position creates a pelvic retroversion which means that the pelvis tilts backwards with a more vertical position of the sacrum. In this situation, the "functional" acetabular anteversion increases (the anterior opening of the acetabulum is greater due to this new posture).

Some subjects have a low sacral tilt angle, even in standing position, which means that the pelvic anteversion is low: we call it "paradoxal pelvic retroversion" and the sacrum seems more vertical on the lateral view of the pelvis. (Fig. 4)

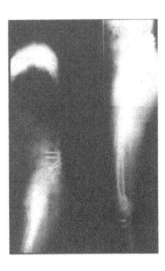

Figure 4:
Lumbosacral arthrodesis with inadequate adjustment
(flat back, vertical sacrum, hips flexion).
On the right view, the patient was asked to correct is
posture as much as possible:
residual hips flexion as the hips don't have sufficient
adaptation possibilities.

Standing with the torso bent forward is inefficient and unstable. The hips and knees flex to compensate and to maintain an upright posture, producing a crouched posture and gait.

This posture puts extra demand on the back extensors, causing fatigue pain. Hip extensor weakness is frequent and the flexion of the hip may serve to place the extensors at a more mechanically advantageous muscle length.

In sitting position, this pelvic retroversion remains or increases. In this case, "functional" acetabular anteversion is abnormally increased and the "Functional Range of Motion" of the hip joint is modified with more internal rotation. This phenomenon has been observed in clinical practice, when studying the gait of patients with spinal fusion inducing a flatback with pelvic retroversion.

On the contrary, some subjects have a very horizontal sacrum in standing position, with a sacral tilt angle more than 50°. In sitting position, the pelvic anteversion remains or slightly reduces. In this case, functional acetabular anteversion is decreased and the "Functional Range of Motion" of the hip joint is deviated to the external rotation.

Lying position (supine)

When the lower limbs are lying in full extension, the anterior pelvic tilt is greater than in standing position. This specific posture can be observed when doing lateral X rays on patients in a dorsal decubitus for a T.H.P. via an anterior approach. This adaptation occurs if the lumbosacral junction is mobile, but, if it is fused or stiff the spatial orientation of the acetabulum can be dramatically modified: this can creates problems for the adaptation of an acetabular implant.

Correlations between lumbo-pelvic sagittal position and acetabular orientation:

Lumbosacral posture influences acetabulum anteversion. Understanding sacral tilt (ST) variations is essential to analyse standing and sitting positions acetabular positions [14].

- For the evaluation of each patient, precise radiological criteria are mandatory. We use full-length lateral radiographs centered on T12 in the standing and sitting positions with a focal film distance of 2 m. The radiographs show the entire trunk, the external acoustic meati, and the upper third of the femurs.

The standing position is standardized as follows: the subject stands in a relaxed position, with the arms folded across the chest to minimize variation due to the effects of trunk posture on the lumbosacral junction. Standardization of the sitting position involves placing the subject with the axes of the thighs perpendicular to the axis of the trunk and no pressure of the trunk against the back of the chair. The subject is asked to remain as relaxed as possible.

Those Xrays allow to measure Sacral Tilt angle (ST); the same measure can be done on classical lateral Xrays, but the same and precise rules must be followed. A classical lateral Xray can be done to appreciate de lying ST angle; this angle can also be measured on CT scan lateral scout view.

The measures of "real" or "functional" acetabular anteversion are realized on CT scan cuts replicating the horizontal planes for the subjects in standing or sitting positions. (Fig. 5)

Conventionnal CT scan evaluation may be inefficient especially when ST standing and ST lying are very different [4] and for the evaluation of sitting position.

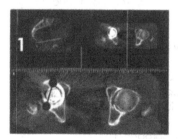
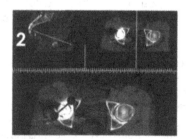
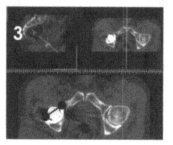

Figure 5:
CT scan measures of « real » or « functional » acetabular anteversion from standing to sitting position. Acetabular anteversion progressively increases.

A CT section plane that goes through femoral head centers and forms with the upper S1 endplate an angle equal to standing ST (measured on the standing film) replicates the horizontal transverse plane in the standing position: it can be used to calculate standing "functional anteversion" of the acetabulum. If an angle equal to sitting ST is used, the plane shows sitting "functional" anteversion of the acetabulum (Sitting ST is usually smaller than standing ST).

- This CT scan technique provides very interesting datas about the real anteversion in usual standing or sitting postures. Additional cuts for different ST angles values (for example every 10°) can also be realized to obtain the global anteversion variations, even in hyperextension or hyperflexion of the lumbosacral area.

- When the range of motion of the spine is normal in the sagittal plane, rotation of the pelvis around a transverse axis gives some room for adjustment during movements of the hip as the normal value for variation of sacral tilt is about 30° between standing and sitting position in our series of control patients. In the standing position, forward rotation of the pelvis uncovers the femoral head posteriorly and improves anterior coverage (marked ST). In the sitting position, the relatively vertical position of the sacrum with backward rotation of the pelvis uncovers the femoral head anteriorly (small ST). Those modifications of sagittal orientation are associated with variations of anatomical anteversion (less cup anteversion in standing position and more cup anteversion in sitting position).

- Diseases affecting the spine or lumbosacral junction (aging spine) and adjustments during prior surgical procedures (lumbosacral fusion) can affect the ST angle. A permanent decrease in ST results in marked anterior uncovering and can cause posterior impingement in the standing position. This situation can occur in patients with degenerative lumbar spine lesions that fix the sacrum in a vertical position in both the sitting and the standing positions. Lumbosacral fusion with a small degree of ST replicating the sitting position can have the same effect.

In patients with limited spinal motion and, in many cases, permanent backward rotation of the pelvis (closed and fixed ST angle), changes in anteversion between the sitting and standing position may be very small. This explains the possible catastrophic consequences of selecting an inappropriate anteversion angle during hip replacement in case of stiff lumbosacral junctions.In such situation, we could observe anterior THP dislocation during hyperextension of the hip in standing position, even in patients implanted via a posterior approach. (Fig. 6)

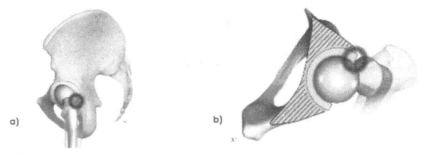

Figure 6:
a) Lateral standing view in a patient with T.H.P. and permanent pelvic retroversion. The potential posterior conflict can be seen. **b)** Idem on a CT scan cut replicating standing position.

On the contrary, we can observe some cases with excessive lumbar lordosis and a very horizontal sacrum. The "functional" acetabular anteversion is low; this particular situation can cause severe problems for T.H.P. acetabular implantation. Actual THP cannot reproduce the real mechanical characteristics and tolerances of normal hip joint. If the only reference is bone architecture and not the dynamic positions of the pelvis, is possible, Low "functional" acetabular anteversion in standing and sitting positions can induce T.H.P. instability.

Walking is associated with changes in the relative anteversion of the acetabular and femoral components. According to the phase in the walking cycle, these changes can result in 5 – 10° of anteversion or retroversion of the femoral component relative to the acetabular cup. When there is little or no femoral component anteversion, relative retroversion can occur if the functional acetabular anteversion in the standing position is inadequate; this can result in impingement or even in dislocation.

But the main instable situation occurs in sitting position, due to anterior impingement. In such cases, we could observe posterior THP dislocations, even in patients implanted via an anterior approach. (Fig. 7)

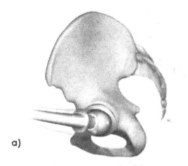
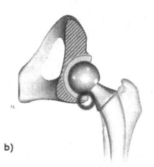

a)

b)

Figure 7:
Patient with T.H.P. and permanent pelvic hyperanteversion.
a) Lateral view in sitting position.
b) On the CT scan cut replicating the sitting position, acetabular anteversion is very low with a potential anterior conflict.

Conclusion

The analysis of sagittal equilibrium of the trunk cannot be limited to the study of spine on lateral Xrays. Hips position and lower limbs adaptation are essential.

Sitting Xrays show very important variations in sagittal equilibrium. All of these Xrays only show "instantaneous" images of complex postural situations.

In-depth knowledge of the mechanics of the lumbosacral junction is essential both for spinal surgeons and for surgeons who perform hip replacements in elderly patients with abnormal sagittal spinal posture and/or a marked reduction in the functional range of motion.

The "pelvic vertebra" adapts the orientation of the each acetabulum, and then, the functional range of motion of the hip joints.

Sagittal sacral tilt is a functional parameter that illustrates the importance of the relationship between pelvis and spine.

It takes into account the extent to which the pelvis can rotate to improve joint motion within the useful range.

In normal subjects ST angle variations are about 30° between standing and sitting position. There is less functional acetabular anteversion in the standing than in the sitting position.

This evaluation of lumbo-pelvic alignment is mandatory for optimization in THP implantation or spinal fusion. (Fig. 8) But those adjustments can be questionable in the future due to progressive changes in postural adaptation of our patients.

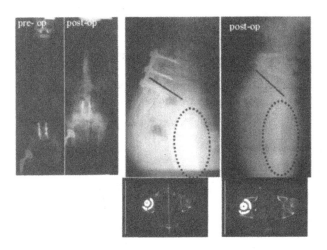

Figure 8: pre-op
Failure of lumbar fusion with major sagittal desequilibrium
- right T.H.P. with permanent adaptative hip flexion
- lumbar pain due to abnormal torse bent posture
- recurrent subluxation of the right T.H.P. due to lack of adaptation possibility in extension (the excessive functional acetabular anteversion in standing position induces an inadapted Functional Range of Motion; posterior impingement in standing position)

post-op
- consequences after lumbosacral fusion correction (wedge osteotomy): permanent hip flexion is reduced and functional acetabular anteversion is corrected in standing position

Pelvic retroversion has decreased and each acetabulum is less anteverted.

References

1. D'Lima D.D., Urquhart A.G., Buehler K.O., Walker R. H., ColwellL C.W.: The effect of the orientation of the acetabular and femoral components on the range of motion of the hip at different head-neck ratios. J. Bone Joint Surg., 82-A, 3, march 2000, 315-321.

2. Dorr L.D., WAan Z.: Causes of and treatment protocol for instability of total hip replacement. Clin Orthop, 355, 1998, 144-151.

3. Duval-Beaupere G. Schmidt C. Cosson P. A Barycentremetric study of the sagittal shape of spine and pelvis: the conditions required for an economic standing position. Annals of Biomedical Engineering. 20(4):451-62, 1992.

4. Eddine TA. Migaud H. Chantelot C. Cotten A. Fontaine C. Duquennoy A. Variations of pelvic anteversion in the lying and standing positions: analysis of 24 control subjects and implications for CT measurement of position of a prosthetic cup. Surgical & Radiologic Anatomy. 23(2):105-10, 2001.

5. Gelb DE. Lenke LG. Bridwell KH. Blanke K. McEnery KW. An analysis of sagittal spinal alignment in 100 asymptomatic middle and older aged volunteers. Spine. 20(12): 1351-8, 1995.

6. Granata KP. Sanford AH. Lumbar-pelvic coordination is influenced by lifting task parameters. Spine. 25(11):1413-8, 2000.

7. Hedlundh U, Karlsson M, Ringsberg K, Besjakov J, Fredin H. Muscular and neurologic function in patients with recurrent dislocation after total hip arthroplasty: a matched controlled study of 65 patients using dual-energy X-ray absorptiometry and postural stability tests. J Arthroplasty. 1999;14:319–25.

8. Itoi E. Roentgenographic analysis of posture in spinal osteoporotics. Spine. 16(7):750-6, 1991.

9. Jackson RP, McManus AC. Radiographic analysis of sagittal plane alignment and balance in standing volunteers and patients with low back pain matched for age, sex, and size. Spine; 19: 1611-8. 1994

10. Korovessis P. Re: Jackson PR, et al. Congruent spinopelvic alignment on standing lateral radiographs of adult volunteers. Spine 2000;25:2808-285.

11. Kummer F.J., Shah S., Iyer S., Di Cesare P.E.: The effect of acetabular cup orientations on limiting hip rotation. J Arthroplasty, 14, 4, 1999, 509-513.

12. Lazennec JY. Saillant G. Saidi K. Arafati N. Barabas D. Benazet JP. Laville C. Roy-Camille R. Ramare S. Surgery of the deformities in ankylosing spondylitis: our experience of lumbar osteotomies in 31 patients. European Spine Journal. 6(4):222-32, 1997

13. Lazennec JY. Ramare S. Arafati N. Laudet CG. Gorin M. Roger B. Hansen S. Saillant G. Maurs L. Trabelsi R. Sagittal alignment in lumbosacral fusion: relations between radiological parameters and pain. European Spine Journal. 9(1):47-55, 2000

14. Lazennec JY, Charlot N, Gorin M, Roger B, Arafati N, Bissery A, Saillant G. Hip-spine relationship: a radio-anatomical study for optimization in acetabular cup positioning. Surgical & Radiologic Anatomy. 25(7), 2003

15. Legaye J. Duval-Beaupere G. Hecquet J. Marty C. Pelvic incidence: a fundamental pelvic parameter for three-dimensional regulation of spinal sagittal curves. European Spine Journal. 7(2):99-103, 1998.

16. Lindberg HO, Carlsson AS, Gentz CF, Pettersson H. Recurrent and non-recurrent dislocation following total hip arthroplasty. Acta Orthop Scand. 1982;53:947–52.

17. Mangione P. Senegas J. [Sagittal balance of the spine]. Revue de Chirurgie Orthopedique et Reparatrice de l Appareil Moteur. 83(1):22-32, 1997

18. Morrey BF. Difficult complications after hip joint replacement dislocation. Clin Orthop. 1997;344:179–87.

19. Nelson JM. Walmsley RP. Stevenson JM. Relative lumbar and pelvic motion during loaded spinal flexion/extension. Spine. 20(2):199-204, 1995

20. Rillardon L. Levassor N. Guigui P. Wodecki P. Cardinne L. Templier A. Skalli W. [Validation of a tool to measure pelvic and spinal parameters of sagittal balance]. Revue de Chirurgie Orthopedique et Reparatrice de l Appareil Moteur. 89(3):218-27, 2003.

20. Sarwahi V. Boachie-Adjei O. Backus SI. Taira G. Characterization of gait function in patients with postsurgical sagittal (flatback) deformity: a prospective study of 21 patients. Spine. 27(21):2328-37, 2002

21. Terver S. Dillingham M. Parker B. Bjorke A. Bleck EE. Levai JP. Teinturier P. Viallet JF. [True orientation of the acetabulum as determined by CAT scan. Preliminary results. Journal de Radiologie. 63(3):167-73, 1982.

22. Tully EA., ; Wagh P.;. Galea MP Lumbofemoral Rythm During Hip Flexion in Young Adults and Children , Spine; 27(20) 432-440 .2002

23. Vedantam R, Lenke LG, Keeney JA, et al. Comparison of standing sagittal spinal alignment in asymptomatic adolescents and adults. Spine; 23: 211-5. 1998

24. Von Knoch M. Berry DJ. Harmsen WS. Morrey BF. Late dislocation after total hip arthroplasty. Journal of Bone & Joint Surgery - American Volume. 84-A(11):1949-53, 2002

25. Woo RY, Morrey BF. Dislocations after total hip arthroplasty. J Bone Joint Surg Am. 1982;64:1295–306

26. Woolson ST, Rahimtoola ZO. Risk factors for dislocation during the first 3 months after primary total hip replacement. J. Arthroplasty, 14, 1999: 662-668

5.3 Design Parameter to Improve Range of Motion (ROM) in Total Hip Arthroplasty

J. Oehy and K. Bider

Introduction

Dislocation represents, after aseptic loosening, the second most frequent complication [1] in total hip arthroplasty (THA) with an occurrence of 2-3% following a primary THA and 10% in revision arthroplasties [2]. Factors contributing to impingement and dislocation include soft tissue, bone components, orientation of the prosthesis, design of the implants [3].
The feasible prosthetic range of motion (ROM) is a function of:
- effective position of the implanted components (influenced by pre- and intra-operative circumstances)
- technical ROM (influenced by the manufacturer's implant design)

It is well recognised that a correctly combined orientation of both components, the acetabular cup and femoral stem, during implantation will yield a maximised ROM and will reduce the risk for dislocation.
However, in current day-to-day clinical practice, even experienced surgeons are not always successful at precisely placing the prosthetic components in relation to one another. As a result of the use of reliable positioning instruments and computer-aided navigation, improvements with regard to the precision of implant positioning may be expected in the future.

The standards for a modern, modular THA have increased in recent years and are intended to provide the patient with good functionality as well as an extended durability within the human body. The mobility and stability that can be achieved following prosthetic treatment in younger, active patients is becoming increasingly more important. For this reason, special care should be taken when designing and choosing the modular prosthetic components to ensure that range of motion and stability are not impaired.

The aim of this paper is to:
- identify general design parameters influencing the technical ROM (T-ROM)
- investigate particular improvements for T-ROM after changes in the design of a femoral stem, femoral head or acetabular cup within the product portfolio of Centerpulse (a Zimmer company)
- discuss the limitations and provide recommendations for desirable component features.

Method

A motion simulation with three-dimensional hip prostheses models was performed using a CAD program (Unigraphics 3D). Based on defined implant positions, the previous prostheses design was compared to new design versions in terms of the maximum range of motion they provide. In each case, the technical range of motion to the point of impingement was determined for individual movements (flexion, extension, abduction, adduction, internal and external rotation).

Following design elements were analysed:
- diameter and design of femoral heads
- neck geometry and taper design for the femoral stem
- design of the entrance plane in the acetabular cup and cup profile.

In addition to these purely kinematic observations, other limiting factors were also discussed.

Results

The attainable technical range of motion to impingement in hip prosthesis models was determined through the use of a 3D-CAD simulation with various geometries in terms of the design of the stem, femoral head and cup.

Diameter and design of femoral heads

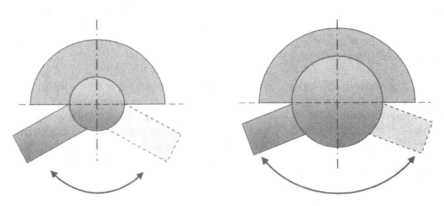

Figure 1:
ROM is a function of femoral head size: An increased articulation diameter dramatically enhances T-ROM.
In addition a larger ratio between femoral head diameter and neck diameter enhances T-ROM.

Many total hip replacements result in limitation of ROM due to of component-to-component impingement. This is particularly true with smaller head sizes and modular femoral heads which require skirts.

Investigations done in this study have uniformly shown an increase in ROM using head sizes of 32 and 36mm, compared to head sizes 28mm or smaller for all four neck lengths. An average increase of 8 and 13 degrees respectively was shown using a 32mm or 36mm femoral head in combination with a standard femoral stem design.

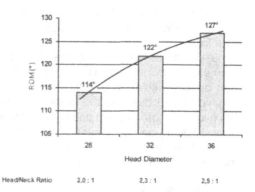

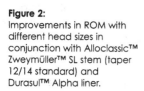
Figure 2:
Improvements in ROM with different head sizes in conjunction with Alloclassic™ Zweymüller™ SL stem (taper 12/14 standard) and Durasul™ Alpha liner.

The femoral head size 28mm XL contains as a result of the longer neck length a cylindrical skirt which reduces maximum possible flexion by about 8 degrees (see Fig. 4). It is recognised that head-neck ratio is an important factor in ROM, primarily due to component-to-component impingement. Larger diameter femoral heads are the most direct way to improve this ratio. Because femoral heads 32mm and larger never require a skirt, regardless of the neck length, the larger heads show a substantial increase in ROM.

On the other hand, the percentage gain in range of motion decreases with increasing head size. This means that the size of the femoral head must be considered, in addition to biomechanical issues, to the number of achievable acetabular liner for the corresponding acetabular components. Anatomy is another limiting factor. Suitable acetabular cups with classic head diameters of 22 or 28 mm are still necessary for very small acetabulum sizes.

Besides enhanced ROM larger femoral heads offer a further distinct advantage: enhanced stability. Larger heads are set deeper into the acetabular liner than the smaller head sizes, thus increasing stability, as they must be displaced further in order to dislocate compared with that of the traditional femoral head sizes. Supporting information confirming the improved stability is available from different in vitro anatomical studies and prior clinical studies in which large femoral heads were used [4,5,6].

Neck geometry and taper design

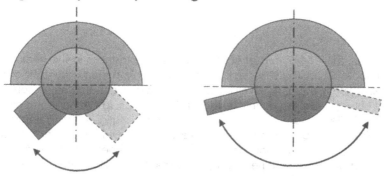

Figure 3:
ROM is a function of neck diameter and taper design: T-ROM increases with decreasing neck diameter.

Early impingement that leads to the generation of debris and possible subsequent dislocation may be caused by a bulky neck diameter or an exposed large taper.

The objective was to evaluate the beneficial effect of a modified neck geometry and taper design with regard to range of motion to impingement. Two stem designs with a taper 12/14 were used, with a major difference in taper length and neck diameter below the taper. Design 1 was a current standard stem with a taper length 14.5mm and a neck diameter 13.5mm. Design 2 had a shorter taper (12.0mm) and a thinner neck diameter (11.6mm).

These two designs were analysed using different head diameters (28-36mm) and neck lengths (-4mm to +8mm).

Results from the computer analysis revealed an average increase in range of motion of 5 degrees.

Shortening the taper length also results in an improvement in ROM especially for head size 28mm L, because the unused lower part of the stem taper is removed, thereby extending the slender part of the slim neck. This measure has no effect on the force of retention of the femoral head on the stem neck, since the minimum bearing taper length remains unchanged.

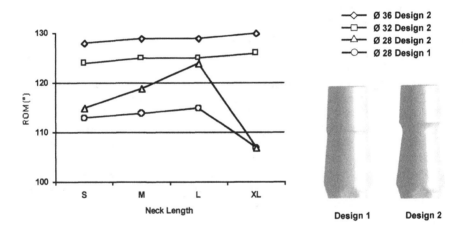

Figure 4:
Improvements in ROM with different neck diameter/taper design in conjunction with various femoral head sizes and neck lengths.

However, the component strength of the stem prosthesis in the neck region does impose limits. The slim neck must also reliably perform the task of load transfer, which is equal to several times the body weight. For this reason, such design changes are thoroughly tested at Centerpulse (a Zimmer company) by means of Finite Element Analyses (FEA) and dynamic fatigue testing before they are implemented. During these tests, it has become evident that the choice of material, production method and design of the prosthetic stem influence the component strength in the neck region and limit the possible extent of reduction of the neck diameter in the slimmer portion.

Design of the entrance plane and cup profile

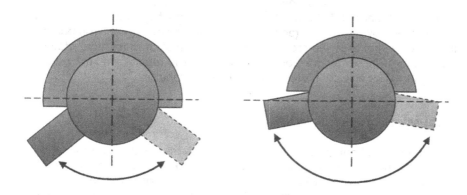

Figure 5:
ROM is a function of the acetabular cup profile: T-ROM increases due to a reduction in the entrance plane of the insert or a reduction of the acetabular cup profile. T-ROM is compromised, at least partly, with the use of hooded inserts.

With any hard-on-hard bearing (metal-on-metal, ceramic-on-ceramic), appropriate positioning of the components is crucial. Neck impingement in a soft-on-hard bearing against a polyethylene insert, although undesirable, is more forgiving with respect to potential damage to the stem or acetabular component.

The aim was to evaluate the beneficial effect with regard to ROM permitted by a slightly modified insert design for the traditional articulation diameter 28 and 32mm. The reason for only a moderate reduction of the entrance plane is to ensure a sufficient coverage of the femoral head by the metallic insert and the resulting stability in vivo.

Design 1 was the existing Metasul Alpha 28mm liner; Design 2 was a Metasul Alpha 28mm liner where the entrance plane of the metallic insert was reduced by 1mm. Design 3 was a Metasul Alpha 32mm liner.

The newly designed Metasul Alpha 28 and 32mm inserts provided improvement with regard to ROM of 7° and 15° respectively.

Figure 6:
Improvements in ROM with slightly modified entrance plane on Metasul™ Alpha liners for two different femoral neck geometries/ taper designs.

Diameter	ROM Std Neck	Head/Neck Ratio	ROM Slim Neck	Head/Neck Ratio
28 std Design 1	114°	2,0 : 1	119°	2,2 : 1
28 opt Design 2	121°	2,0 : 1	126°	2,2 : 1
32 opt Design 3	126°	2,2 : 1	129°	2,4 : 1

A neutral liner should be used wherever possible in order to maximise the impingement-free range of motion. This requires optimal positioning of the metal shell to match the desired orientation of the opening face.

The use of a hooded Metasul Alpha liner shows a substantial reduction in the arc of motion by 10° in the direction of the elevated rim segment compared to that of a neutral liner. This reduction in range of motion makes the rotational positioning of these designs particularly important to reduce rim impingement and potential acceleration of polyethylene wear at the rim.

Discussion

The most important factors influencing post-operative mobility and stability of the artificial hip are the head diameter and the neck geometry, and/or the ratio of head diameter to neck diameter. Increasing the articulation diameter enlarges the range of motion. In addition, stability is increased as a result of the larger femoral head being set deeper into the acetabular cup compared to that of the smaller head sizes. As a result, the risk of impingement is significantly lowered and the risk of dislocation is reduced. However, the use of large femoral heads has only become possible as a result of extremely wear-resistant bearings (metal-on-metal, ceramic-on-ceramic, and highly cross-linked polyethylene), because the wear rates are extremely low, even with large articulation diameters [7, 8, 9].

The literature contains a wide variety of clinical studies on the subject of dislocation, in which the influence of the head diameter was also examined. The clinical results and the consequent benefit with regard to the 22mm to 32mm head diameters in use are subject to controversial discussion. On the one hand, this is due to the wide range of influencing factors, on the other, the authors believe that in the discussion to date, too little attention has been paid to an important parameter: the ratio of head diameter to neck diameter. This ratio is generally not specified in the currently published studies, in spite of the fact that it is precisely this parameter that significantly influences the dislocation rate. In order to obtain a sufficient post-operative hip mobility and stability, total hip endoprostheses should provide a head-neck ratio of at least 2:1 [6]. When determining this ratio, it is important to note that as a result of the neck geometry of the stem, and depending on the selected neck length for the femoral head, the contact point can vary along the neck of femoral stem or can even be at the neck of the femoral head.

Although the influence of the femoral offset on the range of motion was not examined in this study, it also plays an important role. An insufficient offset leads to a loss in soft tissue tension and a reduction in the impingement-free range of motion. A larger, adequate offset offers a number of advantages (Elke, 1998):

- avoids premature bony impingement
- improves the efficiency of the abductors and thereby the gait pattern
- prevents an excessively steep course of the vector of the resulting hip force.

Modern systems for THA should have a minimum range of motion of 120° so as to achieve a satisfactory outcome once implanted. These standards can easily be met and even exceeded by implementing the above mentioned design changes, and by appropriate selection of the components by the physician performing the surgery.

Therefore a recommendation for a modern modular total hip arthroplasty should in future include the following desirable component features:

- use only components which offer a head - neck diameter ratio of at least 2:1
- use largest available femoral head for each cup size
- avoid skirted heads wherever possible
- use femoral stems with favourable neck geometry
- use femoral stems with an adequate offset
- use neutral liners wherever possible.

Summary

Increased range of motion, fewer dislocations - the large femoral heads, an optimised neck geometry at the femoral stem, as well as modification of the acetabular cup profile offer many advantages in modular hip prostheses. In combination with low-wear bearings, the large femoral heads allow an increase in the range of motion, greater stability, and improvement in the durability of artificial hips. However, the optimisation of the individual design elements is also subject to limitations: enlarging the articulation diameter can only be achieved up from a certain acetabular cup size; a narrow neck must continue to perform the function of load transfer without causing fractures in vivo, and a acetabular cup with a reduced entrance plane has to ensure a sufficient coverage of the femoral head. It is therefore important to balance the distribution of measures when implementing any of them into the design of a prosthesis.

References

1. Giurea A et al: Risk factors for dislocation of a cement-free total hip endoprosthesis - a statistical analysis, Z Orthop 2001; 139; 194 - 199
2. Morrey BF: Difficult complications after hip joint replacement. Dislocation. Clin. Orthop. 1997, 344: 179-187
3. Siebenrock KA, Ganz R: The impingement problem in total hip arthroplasty, in: World tribology forum in arthroplasty/Claude Rieker. (ed.) - Berne, Göttingen, Toronto, Seattle: Huber, 2001, 47-52
4. Noble PC, Paravic V, Ismaily S: Are big heads the solution to dislocation after total hip replacement? 48th Annual Meeting of the ORS, 2002, paper 0129
5. Burroughs BR, Rubash HE, Harris WH: Femoral head sizes larger than 32mm against highly cross-linked polyethylene. Clinical Orthopedics and Related Research 405, 2002, 150-157
6. Bader R, Scholz R, Steinhauser E, Mittelmeier W: The importance of prosthesis head design in terms of risk of dislocation following artificial hip replacement - a biomechanical analysis. Orthopädische Praxis 39,7, 2003, 430-435
7. Rieker CR et al: In-vitro tribology of large metal-on-metal implants - influence of the clearance, 50th Annual Meeting of the ORS, 2004, paper 123
8. Saikko V, Pfaff HG: Low wear and friction in alumina/alumina total hip joint: a hip simulator study. Acta Orthop. Scand. 69, 1998, 443-448
9. Muratoglu OK et al: Larger diameter femoral heads used in conjunction with a highly cross-linked ultra-high molecular weight polyethylene. J Arthroplasty 16 (8), Suppl. 1, 2002, 24-30

5.4 Recommendations for Maximizing Range of Motion

J. P. Garino

With the dawn of the new Millennium, Hip replacement surgery entered a new era of expanding indications and technological improvements which seek to further optimize one of the most successful interventions of modern medicine. In the beginning, there was the low friction arthroplasty. John Charnley recognized that synthetic materials did not have the very low wear demonstrated by articular cartilage. For that reason he moved away from the large ball heads that were part of normal human anatomy. Because his technique often resulted in a transposition of the greater trochanter, pain relief and stability along with a protected sedentary lifestyle were the keys to successful outcomes. He was a master at limiting patient expectations and reserving the procedure for the low demand elderly. The leg length discrepancies and other biomechanical alterations were much welcomed trade offs for the comfort and function improvements that were a result of hip replacement. It changed many people's lives. However some 4 decades later, we are faced with a much different situation. Hip replacements are very successful and surprisingly durable. Hip disease in the younger and more active elderly is best treated with this procedure, as no other intervention is able to restore the comfort and function of these patients so reliably. In addition, trauma and osteonecrosis continue to afflict many younger individuals who need to work and raise families. Once again, hip replacement stands alone in its ability to restore comfort and function for the long term.

We have become victims of our own success. With many studies boasting over 95% good to excellent results at 10 years and beyond, surgeons and patients continue to push the activity envelope after hip replacement. Patients undergoing hip replacement surgery are more active than originally thought, with the average patient having over 2 million cycles per year [1]. Polyethylene wear directly correlated with activity, and there is a strong trend toward a much more active elderly population with a long life expectancy. These patients are engaging in activities far more strenuous than just walking. They wish to play with their children or grandchildren (often on the floor), or return to their jobs, many of which are also strenuous. The demands of life, financially and philosophically, are pushing patients to feel more "normal" with their hip replacement, rather than "disabled".

With this in mind, the need for a more functional and durable total hip has developed. With wear the biggest problem faced by surgeons, and polyethylene debris recognized as the main culprit, the standard head size remained at 28mm, a balance between the low volumetric wear but high linear wear of the 22mm ball head and the high volumetric, low linear wear of the 32mm ball head. There was a strong desire to use 32mm ball heads as it represented the smallest size where bony, as opposed to prosthetic impingement was the main source of instability [2]. (Fig. 1) This balance between optimizing wear and stability has always been a difficult one.

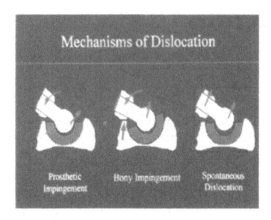

Figure 1a:
Mechanisms of dislocation.

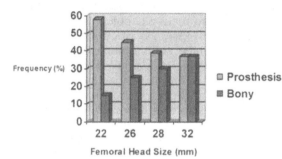

Figure 1b:
Head Size vs. Site of Impingement.

But fortunately, technology continues to modify and improve our devices and with the development of advanced bearings, low wear even for large ball heads is now a reality for both metal-on-metal and ceramic on ceramic systems. Highly-crosslinked polyethylene is also showing some promise in the lab, but longer-term clinical studies are not available and there remain some questions about the amount of crosslinking and subsequent strength reduction of the material. This is particularly true as ball head sizes enlarge, as care must be taken to maintain a sufficient minimum thickness of poly in all areas of the system.

Maximizing the range of motion for optimization of patient function and minimizing instability following total hip replacement therefore has a few key considerations:

      1. Maximizing the size of the ball head.
      2. Using a favorable neck geometry
      3. Avoiding elevated metallic rims on acetabular components
      4. Proper component placement
      5. Choose proper bearing materials
      6. Avoid bone and soft tissue impingement.
      7. Counsel and educate your patient

1. Maximizing the ball head Size. There is no question that the easiest way to improve function and minimize instability in total hip replacement is to eliminate prosthetic impingement of the femoral neck and acetabular component. Studies have shown that the maximum range of motion obtained by any system increases with increasing ball head size [3]. (Fig. 2). In choosing a large ball size,

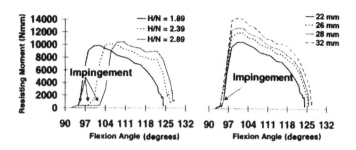

Figure 2:
ROM as a function
of Ball size. [3]

which is now available from multiple manufacturers in 36mm and even 40mm varieties, the bearing surface must be considered. Ceramic on Ceramic systems have some limitations in terms of ball lengths, but the bearing surface has been well investigated over 30 years and remain the lowest wear couple currently available. Risk of ball fracture also decreases with increasing ball head size. The extremely low wear with hard on hard systems eliminates all concerns regarding the theoretical increased volumetric wear with increased ball head sizes [4].

2. Much attention in recent years has been paid by prosthetic manufacturers with respect to optimizing neck geometry for further improvements in range of motion without compromising strength. More trapezoidal geometries with shortened tapers have enhanced this aspect of hip replacements [5]. (fig. 3).

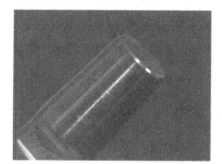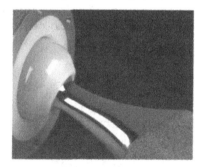

Figure 3:
3a: Old style neck geometries, long and wide.   3b: Streamlined neck geometry example.

3. Any elevation of the cup rim to protect the bearing surface may lead to slightly reduced range of motion as well as mode 4 wear and additional metal debris release if impingement were to occur post-op. With reports of potential problems of these types of designs, consideration for other designs is recommended [6].

4. Proper component placement is by far the most critical aspect of optimizing range of motion. Most studies concur that 45 degrees of flexion is the ideal, balancing the need for significant flexion while limiting wear and stress overload. In addition, anteversion of both the stem and the cup play important roles in optimizing the functional range of motion and stability of the total hip replacement. Femoral anteversion of 15 degrees and acetabular anteversion of 15-30 degrees are also recommended [7]. (Fig. 4). Proper placement of the

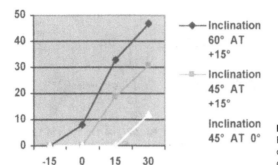

Figure 4:
Range of Motion in internal rotation at 90 degrees of flexion as a function of cup inclination and anteversion.

components has its pitfalls. In the lateral position the patient has an increased lumbar lordosis as the pelvis has a tendency to flex on the table. When it extends in the upright position, there is relatively reduced anteversion. Also, in the lateral position, the pelvis can have a tendency to tip forward, unbeknownst to the surgeon, also resulting in lost anteversion. Trial reduction with trial liner is critical in assessing all-important parameters including leg length, offset and stability. Navigation, or computer assisted surgery, is being developed and reaching the point where it may soon add valuable feed back to the surgeon regarding optimal cup placement.

5. Larger ball heads, as mentioned above, can result in an increased head/neck ratio. This can minimize or eliminate impingement in the normal range of motion zone. However, in order to reduce wear with these larger heads, a hard on hard bearing surface is recommended. Ceramic-ceramic couples have the lowest wear while remaining bio-inert to reduce risks to patients and optimize longevity. (Fig. 5)

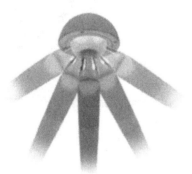

Figure 5:
Increased ROM as a result of larger ball head, improved neck geometry and a ceramic-ceramic couple. (Courtesy of Wright medical technology).

6. Occasionally osteophytes and scar tissue will create impingement points. These tissue impingement points need to be evaluated and reduced with appropriate removal of bone and soft tissue as necessary to minimize this form of impingement.

7. Patient education remains the final key for success. Patients, if they try hard enough, can damage any device that is implanted. Patients must be educated on the limitations of these devices and they should strive to remain within those limitations. Extreme range of motion activities should be discouraged. Patients are encouraged to use their hip replacements, not abuse them.

In Summary, hip replacements continue to evolve and with new techniques and materials, one can continue to meet the increasing demands that are placed on these devices. Proper placement of components coupled with large heads and ceramic bearing materials can optimize the hip replacement for function and longevity for the most active patient.

Reference

1. Schmalzried TP Shepherd EF. Dorey FJ. Jackson WO. dela Rosa M. Fa'vae F. McKellop HA. McClung CD. Martell J. Moreland JR. Amstutz HC. "The John Charnley Award. Wear is a function of use, not time." Clinical Orthopaedics & Related Research. (381):36-46, 2000 Dec.
2. Callaghan, J; Preventing Dislocation: is a big head in your future; Current Concepts in Joint Replacement, Spring 2001.
3. Scifert CF. Brown TD. Pedersen DR. Callaghan JJ. A finite element analysis of factors influencing total hip dislocation. [Journal Article] Clinical Orthopaedics & Related Research. (355):152-62, 1998 Oct et al. Clin Orthop 1998
4. Mckellop H, Lu B. Friction, lubrification, and wear of cobalt-chromium, alumina, and zirconia hip prostheses compared on a joint simulator. Proc. Orthopedic Research Society, Washington, D.C. 402, 1992.
5. Barrack RL. Dislocation after total hip arthroplasty: implant design and orientation. Journal of the American Academy of Orthopaedic Surgeons. 11(2):89-99, 2003 Mar-Apr.
6. Gustafson, A; Clarke I, "metalosis of ceramic-ceramic THR secondary to rim impingement", Bioceramics in Joint Arthroplasty, edited by H. Zippel, M. Dietrich, Steinkopff Verlag, 2003.
7. Bader R. Steinhauser E. Gradinger R. Willmann G. Mittelmeier W. [Computer-based motion simulation of total hip prostheses with ceramic-on-ceramic wear couple. Analysis of implant design and orientation as influence parameters]. [German] [Journal Article] Zeitschrift für Orthopädie und Ihre Grenzgebiete. 140(3):310-6, 2002 May-Jun.

5.5 THA Ceramic-Ceramic Coupling: The Evaluation of the Dislocation Rate with Bigger Heads

L. Zagra, R. Giacometti Ceroni and M. Corbella

Summary

According to Charnley, the rationale to reduce the head diameter in THA is in decreasing the friction torque and the volumetric wear, but, employing a ceramic-ceramic coupling instead of a metal-polyethylene one, bigger diameters can be used without increasing in a considerable way neither the volumetric wear rate nor the friction torque.

The rationale of this study is to evalue if, using a bigger diameter head, the artificial joint is more stable.

In the last two and half years a new acetabular component, with 36 mm liner head alumina-alumina coupling, has been developed and implanted.

We performed a randomized perspective study to investigate the rate of dislocation of the prostheses in the first three months after operation. We matched two cohorts groups, comparable in diagnosis and age, in which the surgical technique (postero-lateral approach), the surgeons, the neck geometry and the off-set of the stem were the same.

In the first one (225 cases, from March 2001 to December 2002) 36 mm heads were implanted, and in the second one (151 cases, from January 2001 to December 2002), 28 mm heads were used. We compared the number of dislocations: 2 (0.88%) in the first group and 7 (4.64%) in the second.

The data confirmed that there is a statistically significant (p=0.02) dislocations decrease in the 36 mm heads group.

Introduction

Concerning hip arthroplasty, throughout the years, many different proposals of head diameters and coupling were made. Charnley was the first that demonstrated the need to reduce the diameter of the femoral heads to decrease the friction torque and the volumetric wear rate [1], which are fundamental for the prosthesis survival. That is true for the metal-polyethylene coupling and it is also partially true for the ceramic-polyethylene coupling [2]. The head diameter reduction was possible only at the cost of a reduction of the joint stability and consequent increase of the dislocation risk [3, 6].

In the meantime the ceramic-ceramic coupling had a progressive diffusion thanks to its lower friction coefficient and to its higher wear resistance [2]. The ceramic is an inert material with high biotolerability [7]. After some initial failures that depended to either the errors of heads and necks design ("skirt heads") [8] or to the fact that the bone doesn't ingrow the ceramic [2], this material has shown to be reliable also in the ceramic-ceramic coupling if used, as a liner, in a metal cup. The ceramic risk fracture, thanks to the tecnological research, is very low and the belated loosening due to the ceramics stiffness are not reported [9, 14].

The 28 mm diameter heads have been the most used till now.

If the neck geometry remains the same, it is possible to increment the joint movement and stability by increasing the head diameter [3,15,16]. That's because, with this standard, the angle to which the neck comes into conflict with the cup rim (Fig. 1), and the distance that the head must cover before getting out of the liner are increased (Fig. 2).

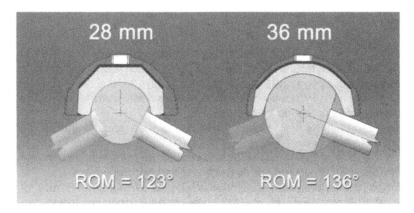

Figure 1:
Increased range of motion (with the same geometry of the neck).

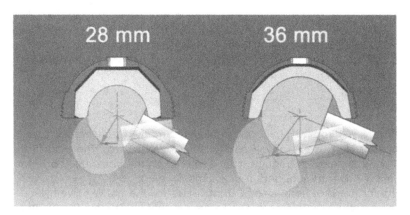

Figure 2:
More difficult dislocation.

With a ceramic-ceramic coupling, the diameter of the head can be increased because, during physiological loads, the friction torque (M=friction moment), thanks to the lower friction coefficient of the ceramic, doesn't significantly get higher (Fig. 4). Reducing the friction torque, proportional to the head radius (r) and the friction coefficient (μ), as focused by Charnley [1], means decreasing the shear forces at the bone-cup interface (Fig. 3). These forces are described in this way:

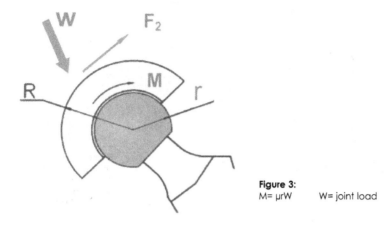

Figure 3:
M= µrW   W= joint load

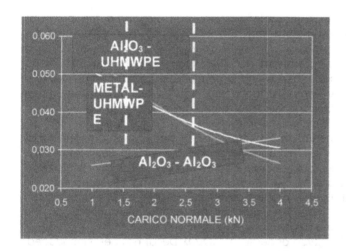

Figure 4:
Friction coefficient
in a range of
standard loads
(Dalla Pria 1998).

Increasing the head diameter from 28 to 36 mm the friction torque gets higher of a factor of 1.29 times; since the ceramic-ceramic friction coefficient is inferior of 1.33 times than the metal-polyethylene, the friction torque doesn't increase.

Although the wear debris is proportional to the head diameter. If we consider that the linear wear (mm/year) is quite constant for any head diameter, the volume of wear (V) can roughly be written:

$$V= \pi r^2 \times Linear\ wear$$

If we increase the head diameter from 28 to 36 mm, in the metal-polyethylene or ceramic-polyethylene coupling, there is an increase of the volumetric wear rate of 2.6 times (Fig. 5), while in the ceramic-ceramic coupling there is an increase wich is lower of almost 100 times than the metal/ceramic-polyethylene one.

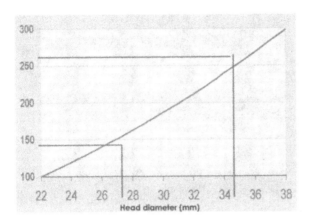

Figure 5:
Volumetric wear
rate related to the
head diameter
(UHMWPE-metal).

Thanks to the material characteristics, we can overcome the problems described by Charlney, even if they still maintain all their validity making problematic to use big heads with other coupling [17]. In this way, using a ceramic-ceramic coupling instead a conventional polyethylene there is no need to use small diameter heads and large diameter heads can give us only benefits without disavantages. At the actual state of technology the 36 mm diameter, for the ceramic, is the ideal compromise between optimal head dimensions and liner safety.

According to these theoretical statements, a new acetabular component that uses liners in ceramic for 36 mm heads has been projected [15, 18]. It is used in a titanium press-fit cup. The cup is porous coated; the primary stability is improved by fins which are parallel to the equator and it could be increased with the addition of screws. The ceramic of the liner is alumina with a cone angle of 18°, higher than the ones currently used, that makes the introduction and the extraction more easy and safety.

In the last year a new type of ceramic (BIOLOX®Delta) has been introduced. This ceramic has a possibility of fracture 12 times inferior than the alumina. That makes possible to produce liners with a small thickness (36 mm for at least 50 mm cups and 32 mm at least 44 mm cups) with higher safety and very small risks of fracture.

The aim of these study is to compare the risk of dislocation, after hip arthroplasty, in two homogeneus (numerically, age, diagnosis, operators and surgical technique) groups of patients; the first with 36 mm diameter ceramics heads and the second with 28 mm diameter heads.

Patients and Methods

We compared 2 randomized groups of patients: a perspective consecutive series of primary hip arthroplasty with 36 mm diameter heads and another one with 28 mm heads, in order to verify the number of dislocations in the first three months after the surgical operation. The neck geometry and the off-set of the stem were the same. The two groups were also homogeneous for patients age, operators (R.G.C., C.P., L.Z.), surgical technique (postero-lateral approach with capsular and external-rotator muscles reconstruction) and post-operative treatment (bed position with abduction pillow between the legs, beginning of walking in the second day with 2 crutches). There was not a complete pre-operative diagnosis homogeneity. In fact in the second group the fractures are more numerous. We don't know if this element determines modifications of the dislocation risk, but it doesn't seem so [6, 19].

The first group is composed of 225 cases of 36 mm heads (from March 2001 to December 2002): mean age 64 years and 9 months, 83 males and 142 female. Diagnosis: 175 degenerative arthritis, 25 DDH, 16 femoral neck fractures, 4 post-traumatic arthritis, 2 SA, 4 femoral head necrosis, 1 Paget disease.

The second group was of 151 cases of 28 mm heads (from January 2001 to December 2002): mean age 66 years, 44 males and 107 female. Diagnosis: 92 degenerative arthritis, 26 DDH, 30 femoral neck fractures, 3 post-traumatic arthritis.

For the statistic analysis we used the chi-square-test.

Results

In the group with 36 mm heads there were 2 dislocations (0.88%) in two male patients: the first was an anterior sub-dislocation reduced with a close reduction in a patient with DDH and the second required an open reduction in a patient with a severe post-traumatic arthritis. There were no recurrent dislocations.

In the 28 mm heads group the dislocations were 7 (4.63%), 5 females and 2 males. This percentage is not very different than the ones reported by other Authors [20, 6]. The diagnosis were: 2 primary arthritis, 2 DDH and 3 fractures. Again, we don't know if the number of fractures, higher in the second group, is significant. We intend to increase the number of patients to eliminate this discrepancy. In all the cases a close reduction was performed. 4 had not further dislocation episodes. In the three cases in which there were recurrent dislocations we proceeded to a substitution of the head with 10.5 mm neck (diagnosis of femur neck fracture), to a substitution of the cup that was excessively antiverse (in a case of dysplasic arthritis) and to a total revision with 36 mm head (in a primary arthritis)

These results show a significant reduction of the dislocation risk in the group of patients operated with 36 mm diameter heads (0.88% versus 4.63% in those with 28 mm heads). This difference is statistically significant (chi^2 = 5,42 - p= 0.02) and it confirms the theoretical assumptions from which the study departed.

	Cohort 1		Cohort 2	
	cases	**dislocations**	**cases**	**dislocations**
Degenerative arthritis	175	0	92	2
DDH	25	1	26	2
Fracture	16	0	30	3
Post-traumatic arthritis	4	1	3	0
(Necrosis, SA)	5	0	0	0

Discussion

According to this study, we could assert that the theoretical lower dislocation risk of hip arthroplasty with coupling of larger diameter, is confirmed in the clinical evidence.

The alumina-alumina coupling with heads of bigger diameter doesn't significantly increase the wear and the friction torque and therefore it is possible to use 36 mm diameter heads increasing the stability and the joint excursion.

The 36 mm heads can be use for cups of 50 mm and greater; while for the 44, 46 and 48 mm cups the head diameter is 32 mm. That makes possible an extension of the indications, a reduction of the dislocations, a better biocompatibility and resistance. The disadvantages depend on the fact to introduce a new standard with an increase of the stock and consequently the possibility of error, particularly in case of partial revisions; but 36 mm is becoming the new standard for big diameter heads.

References

1. Charnley J. Low friction arthroplasty of the Hip. Berlin Heidelberg New York: Springer-Verlag 1979
2. Willmann G. The evolution of ceramics in total hip replacement. Hip Int 2000; 10: 193-203
3. Bartz RL, Nobel PC, Kadakia NR, Tullos HS. The effect of femoral component head and acetabular size to the prevalence of dislocation. J Bone J Surg Am 2000; 82: 1300-7
4. Kelley SS, Lachiewicz PF, Hickman JM, Paterno SM. Relationship of femoral head and acetabular size to the prevalence of dislocation. Clin Orthop 1998 Oct; 335:163-70
5. Hedlundh U, Ahnfelt L, Hybbinette CH, Wallinder L, Weckstrom J, Fredin H. Dsilocations and femoral head size in primary total hip arthroplasty. Clin Orthop 1996; 333:226-33
6. Yuan L, Shih C. Dislocation after total hip arthroplasty. Arch Orthop Trauma Surg 1999, 119: 263-6
7. Lerouge S, Huk O, Yahia L, Witvoet J, Sedel L. Ceramic-ceramic and polyethylene total hip replacement: comparison of pseudomembranes after loosening. J Bone J surg Br 1997; 79:135-9
8. Fritsch EW, Gleitz M. Ceramic femoral head fractures in total hip arthroplasty. Clin Orthop 1996; 328:129-36
9. Sedel L. Evolution of alumina-on-alumina implants: a review. Clin Orthop 2000; 379:48-54
10. Toni A, Terzi S, Sudanese A, Bianchi G. Fractures of ceramic components in total hip arthroplasty. Hip int. 2000;10:49-56
11. Toni A, Sudanese A, Paderni S, Guerra E. Ceramic-on-Ceramic: Long-term clinical experience. Bioceramics in Joint Arthroplasty. Stuttgart: Georg Thieme Verlag 2001: 2-5
12. Boheler M, Knahr K, Plank H, Walter A, Salzer N, Schiriber V. Long term results of uncemented alumina acetabular implants. J Bone J Surg Br 1994; 76: 53-9
13. Garcia-Cimbrelo E, Sayanes, JM Minuesa. Ceramic-ceramic prosthesis after 10 years. J Arthroplasty 1996; 11: 773-81
14. Gualtieri G, Nirgrisoli M, Dallari D, Catamo L, Gualtieri I. A study of the mechanical and biological behaviour of bioceramic hip arthroplasty followed up after more than 10 years. Chir Organi Mov 1993; 78:213-22.
15. Giacometti Ceroni R., Dalla Pria P. The development of large ceramic heads to obtain more stable THA with wider range of motion. Bioceramics in Joint Arthroplasty. Stuttgart: Georg Thieme Vergal 2001: 11-2

16. Yamaguchi M, Akisue T, Bauer TW, Hashimoto Y. The spatial location of impingement in total hip arthroplasty. J Arthroplasty 2000; 15: 305-13

17. Nessutt R, Wimmer MA, Schneider E, Morlock MM. The influence of resting periods on friction in the artificial hip. Clin Orthop 2003; 407: 127-38

18. Zagra L, Marciano E, Giacometti Ceroni R. Alumina-on-alumina coupling with 36 mm heads. Hip Int 2002; 12:200

19. Khan MA, Brakenbury PH, Reynolds ISR. Dislocation following total hip replacement. J Bone J Surg Br 1982; 63:214-8

20. Cabanela ME. Is the posterior approach to THA a choice for all season. Orthopedics 2000; 23: 422

Ceramics in Orthopaedics

The deciding move in hip replacement – BIOLOX®

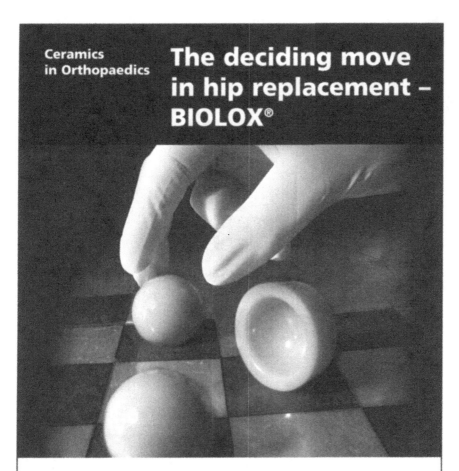

BIOLOX® has excellent biocompatibility and excellent wear resistance.
It is number one in tribology due to its excellent surface properties.
For the patient it offers excellent quality of life and excellent performance.
And you can be sure of BIOLOX®, because its performance has been
proven in clinical use. Yet BIOLOX® offers the way forward for the future.
It sets new standards in orthopaedic applications.

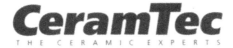

CeramTec
THE CERAMIC EXPERTS

CeramTec AG
Innovative Ceramic Engineering
Medical Products Division
Fabrikstraße 23-29
D-73207 Plochingen
Tel. +49 7153 611 828
Fax +49 7153 611 838
medical_products@ceramtec.de
www.biolox.de